30.3 human factors
40.2

DYNAMIC RESEARCH, INC.

PLEASE RETURN
TO LIBRARY

VEHICLE PERFORMANCE
Understanding Human Monitoring and Assessment

VEHICLE PERFORMANCE

Understanding Human Monitoring and Assessment

Edited by

J. P. Pauwelussen

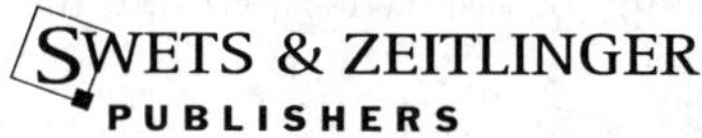

SWETS & ZEITLINGER
PUBLISHERS

LISSE ABINGDON EXTON (PA) TOKYO

Library of Congress Cataloging-in-Publication Data

Applied for

Cover design: Paula van der Heijdt
Printed in the Netherlands by Krips, Meppel

ISBN 90 265 1542 1

CONTENTS

Foreword

Vehicle manufacturers presently put increasing demands on the various parts of a vehicle in order to guarantee optimal vehicle handling, comfort and safety qualities as envisaged in the vehicle design. Since most of the verification of vehicle performance qualities is based on human judgement, a better understanding of the driver monitoring and assessment process will contribute to an improved vehicle-driver response and a more efficient and effective design process. In particular, this is true when the additional benefits of introducing advanced control concepts as part of new designs are considered, with the object of establishing a high level of comfort and to improve or maintain the safety of the vehicle under a wide range of driving conditions.

The success of critical automotive component design from an engineering, marketing or business point of view, is based to a large extent upon this human judgement of vehicle handling and driving qualities. The subjective nature of such evaluation implies business risks for manufacturers when investing in these developments. It puts limits on the effectiveness of their efforts to control and rationalise the vehicle performance improvement process. This situation may be improved by dissemination of the-state-of-the art knowledge of how to link human assessment of vehicle performance to objective vehicle characteristics, and identify the missing links in this interdisciplinary field of international concern.

The seminar **Understanding Human Monitoring and Assessment** was devoted to these issues with, as a central theme, the understanding why a driver judges something good or bad and how this has to be translated into reproducible experiments. This includes not only handling behaviour but also comfort and noise since these aspects contribute to the assessment of vehicle performance by the driver. It was hosted in Delft, Holland, from 20 to 21 November 1997 by the TNO Road-Vehicles Research Institute, organised together with the Delft University of Technology. It was sponsored by the European Community Programme LEONARDO through the EUROMOTOR European Motor Industry Training Network.

Over two days, experts in their fields presented both a broad and in-depth outline of the fields of rationalisation of human judgement in three sessions, reported in this book. Among them is a survey by Cristoph Jung and Wolfgang Hirschberg of recent developments in the field of driver support under particular consideration of the requirements of commercial vehicles, with emphasis on on-line identification of the payload and its position as important parameters with respect to the vehicle's driving behaviour. Two papers have been presented on monitoring and assessment of drivers with special needs, by Björn Peters and Aleid Hekstra et. al., respectively. The first one investigates the use of a driving simulator to establish subjective workload and control of drivers with disabilities. The paper by Aleid Hekstra and

Rinus Kempeneers demonstrates that vehicle design principles which are still based on "average" physical abilities of the user need to be reconsidered in view of a growing elderly and disabled population.
An example how to account for human behaviour in the design of active control elements is dealt with by Wolfgang Kiesewetter et. al. based on the new brake assist active driver support in emergency braking situations.

Three contributions are included on methodologies. Robin Sharp describes the various vehicle qualities in relation to human judgement. Alexander de Vos and Hans Godthelp give a full account of subjective and objective assessment techniques with respect to manual, supported and automated vehicle control. A method of constructing sensitivity functions based on response variables such as yaw rate, side-slip and roll angle is described by Arvin Savkoor, Hugo Happel and François Horkay. The basis of sensitivity functions and correlation-studies between subjective rating and objective monitoring are treated by myself with focus on the effect of tyre handling characteristics on driver assessment. This topic is treated as well by Paul Stephens in his contribution on the influence of the tyre on subjective handling. The seminar has been closed by two interesting contributions touching ride comfort and noise, respectively. Detlef Kudritzki presents a design concept including the necessary analysis for assessment of ride comfort. Dave Fish explains some of the typical psycho-acoustic phenomena experienced in vehicles during normal vehicle operation, and the methods used to interpret vehicle occupant response to noise.

The aim of the seminar was to be an introductory course focusing on the general field of human judgement of vehicle performance, with relevant technologies to be presented in a basic fundamental way within a multidisciplinary framework. It was evident that this seminar fully served its purpose. There appeared to be quite some interest with a large number of representatives of automotive industries being present. Various points of view have been discussed in the seminar as originating from the fields of vehicle technology, human factors, advanced control, etc. The point of view of the design engineer, expert driver, driver with special needs have been addressed. Both applications and methodologies (correlation studies, derivation of appropriate criteria) have been touched on. This approach enabled attendees with various backgrounds to understand the needs, problems and language of their colleagues from different disciplines, and to put the topic of understanding human monitoring and assessment in a broad perspective.

The seminar **Understanding Human Monitoring and Assessment** has been a very fruitful event, with many interesting in-depth discussions at the interface of different disciplines and backgrounds. Last but not least, it was also an enjoyable event due to the highly appreciated operational management by Jolanda Duyvesteyn.

J.P.PAUWELUSSEN
Delft, The Netherlands, September 1998

Session:

Driver Support

Vehicle Performance: J.P. Pauwelussen (ed.) pp. 3-23 © Swets & Zeitlinger

Payload Monitoring as One Basis for Commercial Vehicles Dynamics

Christoph Jung and Wolfgang Hirschberg

The paper gives a survey over recent developments in the field of driver support under particular consideration of the requirements of commercial vehicles. These research activities have been carried out by MAN Nutzfahrzeuge AG.

The paper mainly deals with on-line identification of the payload and its position as important parameters with respect to the vehicle's driving behaviour.

Firstly, the basic correlations between the stability limits due to braking potential, lane keeping and rolling over are discussed. Thus, in contrast to passenger cars, the full three-dimensional stability problem can be shown. The available input quantities for proper vehicle handling are summarized, as well as the influence of active or semiactive subsystems to these properties.

In principle, the driver is responsible for keeping the correct payload according to the legal limitation. For proper vehicle handling of trucks and truck/trailer combinations respectively, the driver also has to fit the driving speed with respect to the current payload and the suitable lateral acceleration. Additionally, the height of CG of payload above ground is a further important safety parameter for roll over warnings. Particularly vehicles with air suspension offer appropriate possibilities to estimate these parameters in a very accurate manner. Furthermore, the amount and position of payload represent additional input suitable for any safety-relevant active subsystem, such as Electronic Brake Systems and Vehicle Stability Controllers.

1. INTRODUCTION

The transportation sector tends to require continuously vehicles with higher technical performance and more and more sophisticated solutions for increasing transportation efficiency and quality. One basic reason for this tendency is the increasing amount of high-valued goods and the high time constraints in transportation, which are beside others due to just-in-time and system-supplying production concepts in the manufactoring world.

Modern truck development takes this into account by introducing optimized vehicles with best handling characteristics and additional comfort and safety features like ABS, improved air suspensions (ECAS), Electronic Damper Control (EFR), Electronic Brake Control and Anti Slip Devices (EBS,ASR), Electronic Power Steering (Servotronic), Adaptive Cruise Control (ACC) and so on.

On the other hand accident statistics are showing that most of all accidents happen because of drivers errors. Looking at accident analysises related to the lateral dynamic of commercial vehicles one will find the following main reasons for leaving the road:

- sudden course deviation, often in combination with braking and a too high initial speed
- too high curve speed

- getting on the unfortified banquet
- wrong estimation of the actual road condition and friction value
- drivers falling asleep
- a moving load

Each of these reasons may be sufficient for causing an accident but in many cases there will occure a combination of them.

To improve driving stability one of the basic information for the driver and subsequent control systems is the knowledge of the actual loading condition with the full three-dimensional position of the centre of gravity.

The following paper gives a survey over recent developments in this field carried out by MAN Nutzfahrzeuge AG during the last years.

1.1 Range of Vehicle Parameters

Looking at commercial vehicles one is faced with a numerous amount of different vehicle types like tractor/trailer and tractor/semitrailer combinations, vehicles with cargo decks, boxbody vehicles, container carriers, tippers, customer built assemblies, bonetrucks and so on optimized for special transportation needs. Beside this large amount of vehicle variations even the parameters of one vehicle can vary very much. Between unloaded and loaded vehicle there is for example a band width from 7,5 to 40 t gross vehicle weight for semitrailer combinations or 9 to 26 t for container carriers.

In comparison to passenger cars, where the payload is at maximum 30% of total vehicle weight, the wide range of loading conditions will result in heavy changes in vehicle driving behaviour and stability characteristics which may not be quite obvious for the driver at the beginning of a ride.

Changes in total mass will result in different longitudinal dynamics of the truck and therefore be discernible and within limits evident for the driver. But even looking at actual axle loads and the margin to their legal limits it becomes quite difficult for the driver to calculate the correct values. So much the more it will be more difficult for him to rate the complete loading status with respect to the height of the centre of gravity, which may vary between 1,1 meter for a partly loaded vehicle and may end up at 2 meters or more under worst case conditions for the fully loaded truck.

- Wheel base and roll centre height
- roll stiffness
- spring and damper tuning

and load dependent values like:

- total mass and centre of gravity
- momentum of inertia of loading.

Figure 1 shows the bandwidth of possible positions of the centre of gravity (CG) due to tolerable front and rear axle loads.

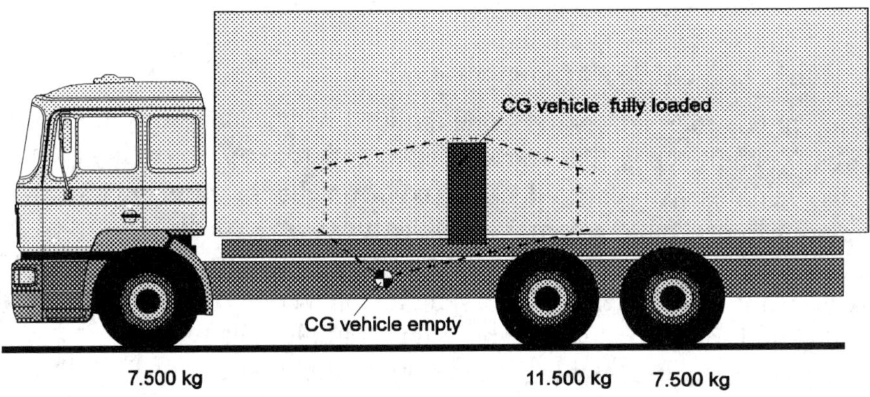

Figure 1: Range of tolerable CG

Beside this tolerable range there exists a wider range as a result of daily loading reality depending on loading and unloading stops.

The limits of maximum tolerable lateral accelerations vary between 2-3 m/s^2 with respect to not fixed goods, 3-4 m/s^2 for bulk goods up to 6-6,5 m/s^2 as rollover limit for modern truck/trailer combinations with low to normal height of centre of gravity and nearly stationary longitudinal and lateral acceleration conditions. Exceptional cases result particularly for higher CGs and moving goods with limits between 3-5 m/s^2. In these special cases, where vehicle reactions may occur quite suddenly and unexpected for the driver, information on loading conditions, warnings and

Especially with the increasing number of container transports the relevance and need of additional information and warnings for the driver may rise due to the lack of information on the stacking of the goods inside.

1.2 Loading of Commercial Vehicles

The following types of loading can be distinguished:

- mixed goods without additional fixation
- paletted goods
- dispatch boxes (ready made, fixed or loose)
- lying or stacked goods without fixation
- stacked goods with fixation (single or double level trailers)
- hanging goods
- containers with unknown load distribution
- bulk material
- fluids or gas in tanks
- moving goods (concrete mixers, animals, etc.)

All these different kinds of vehicle loading can't normally be influenced by the driver and make it necessary for him to adapt his speed and driving style.

Concerning the influence on the vehicle dynamics we have to distinguish the following basic characteristics:

1. Limit of maximum tolerable lateral acceleration determined by danger of load damage or loss of goods

2. Risk of rollover due to exceeded lateral acceleration determined by maximum lateral vehicle stability and actual road conditions (friction limits)

3. Latent risk of rollover triggered by inherent dynamics of loading

As regards item 2, the rollover stability of the vehicle can be described by the following vehicle parameters which are also given in figure 2 and will be discussed later on:

in some cases active controller reactions are to be aspired in time before
critical situations occur. On the other hand this leads to high demands on
the quality of the payload monitoring system.

1.3   Driver Responsibilities

Before starting the ride the driver has the responsibility to check the
proper vehicle condition (brakes, lights, tyre pressures, engine status
etc.). Moreover, he is obliged to check the payload, the total weight and
has to ensure that the maximum axle loads are not exceeded.
For this duty he can make use of the freight papers and weight declara-
tions and if available he may drive on a weighbridge.

For estimating the vehicle´s dynamics he will get some information out
of the handling characteristics while driving which gives him an idea of
the loading condition, especially the eccentricy and height of the centre
of gravity.

All these informations will help the driver to adapt his speed to the road
and traffic conditions with respect to vehicle handling limits and braking
potential.

1.4   Driving Stability

The term "driving stability" is usually defined as a general characteristic
of a driver-vehicle-road system, where "the vehicle is to stay within a
given driving state at any time". The borders of this area are given by the
lane itself and by the road users, as well as by possible obstacles. The
vehicle's dynamical state $\mathbf{x}(t)$ is described by its current position and ve-
locities.

For commercial vehicles, particularly for heavily loaded trucks, there
exists a further stability failure in terms of overturning. This reason of
stability loss is closely related to the remaining longitudinal and lateral
motions of the vehicle so that *all* motions have to be taken into account at
the same time. Due to this fact any simplified investigations in pure lateral dynamics are no longer useful. Contrary to the efforts in passenger
car's dynamics the full spherical consideration and modelling of trucks is
required for advanced driving dynamics.

Hence, any early information and advice on safety-margin-related issues may help the driver to start the appropriate driving operations to maintain the stability and controllability of the truck at any time.

The input quantities necessary for a successful and predicting driving stability evaluation can in principle be classified as

    a) Vehicle motions $\mathbf{x}(t)$
    b) Friction $\mu(s)$
    c) Geometrical road properties

where a fixed relation between the time t and the distance s exists.

Generally, the vehicle's motions depend on the vehicle's dynamical parameters in addition to the disturbation and control inputs.

Typically of commercial vehicles, the payload mass m_L and its position vector $\mathbf{p}_L$ (particularly its height coordinate h_L) have a strong influence on the stability margin. This is why a reliable driving state estimator requires in practice the automatic identification of payload at the beginning of each drive.

ad a) Vehicle motions
Concerning the motions of a commercial vehicle we have to distinguish between
- variables with direct influence on stability margin and
- additional dynamical variables as input into the observer (for state observation use only).

Not all of these time dependent quantities can be measured under practical (serial) conditions. However, the following signals are well qualified for a reliable on-board monitoring:

Wheel speeds ω_i, i=1, 2 ... N_{wh} (available from ABS signal)

Longitudinal and lateral chassis acceleration a_x', a_y',
where ' refers to chassis fixed coordinates

Relative roll angles $\Delta\phi_f$, $\Delta\phi_r$ between axles and frame
where f stands for front, r is for rear

Yaw velocity ω_z
Steering wheel angle δ_S

The remaining properties of interest such as the

Dynamical wheel loads F_{zi} , i=1, 2 ... N_{wh}

are hardly measurable. Therefore they better are estimated by means of a dynamical state observer.

Any autonomous on-board monitoring/estimation system operating by the observation of the vehicle's **dynamical reactions** can only perform a short term prediction of the ongoing dynamical process.

ad b) Friction monitoring
Autonomous friction monitoring systems provide at best a **snap-shot-information** on the current road-tire contact. Any further predetermination of friction-related warnings needs an input from an external host (environmental service).

However, the latter must be considered as a longterm goal of realization due to the necessary fine degree of resolution of fast changing friction data over all the supported roads. One can resume that the only realistic alternative in friction detection is restricted to an autonomously working friction monitoring system (or a combination of existing systems) in the near future.

ad c) Geometrical road properties
The predictive information on the geometrical lane trends

Road slope $\beta(s)$
Road inclination $\alpha(s)$
Road curvature $R(s)$

are important input quantities for any correct information on a proper driving mode (also see below). This information can be available from a digital road map, which is nowadays common for in-vehicle navigation systems.

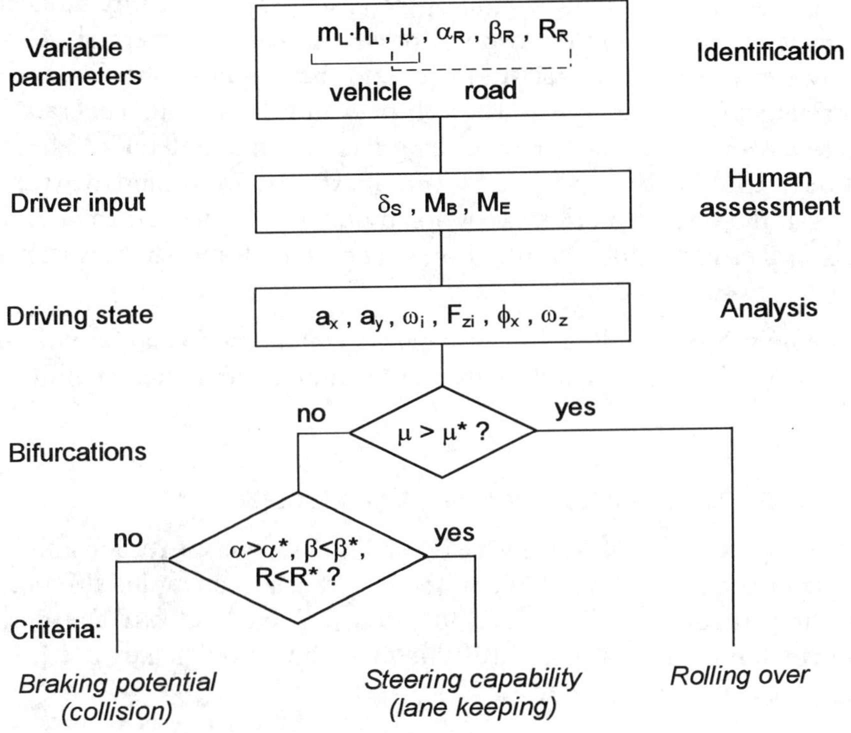

Figure 2: Basic scheme of the driving stability of commercial vehicles

Notations:

m_L	mass of payload	a_x	longitud. acceleration
h_L	height of payload	a_y	lateral acceleration
μ	road-tyre friction	ω_i	angular wheel speeds
α_R	lateral road inclination	F_{zi}	dynamic wheel loads
β_R	longitudinal road slope	ϕ_x	roll angle
R_R	curve radius	ω_z	yaw rate
δ_S	steering angle		
M_E	engine torque		
M_B	braking torque		

Figure 2 shows the discrimination of the basic driving stability modes for commercial vehicles. In opposite to passenger cars commercial vehicles will roll-over at high lateral speeds due to the height of the CG and the characteristics of their tyres. The roll-over thresholds will generally lay between 4 and 6,5 m/s^2. Not exceeding this maximun lateral acceleration the next criteria for losing stability will be the maximum deliverable forces at the tyre splitted between longitudinal and lateral demand. This leads to the distinctions between braking potential and steering capability.

All future vehicle stabilization systems for commercial vehicles will have to provide this discrimination between the above mentioned stability criteria.

2.   DRIVER ASSESSMENT FOR SAFE TRANSPORT

The transport of heavy loads transfers a high amount of responsibility to the driver. As already pointed out, the driver has to adapt his driving behaviour particularly with regard to the actual payload *and* the current road conditions. In order to fulfil this task, the driver makes use of the following main input quantities:

- Visual:

  - Vehicle speed
  - Roll and yaw angle
  - Vehicle position and distance
  - Road geometry

- Audio-visual:

  - Texture of road and weather
  - External and internal warnings

- Haptic:

  - Steering angle and steering torque needed

- Kinaesthetic:

  - Longitudinal, lateral and vertical acceleration
  - Yaw acceleration.

In contrast to the assessment of the road and weather conditions, there is no direct sensor for the actual magnitude and position of the payload except some a priori informations (if available so far). Thus, the experience of the driver allows the more or less good estimation of the payload and its position based upon the above listed observations.

On the other hand, more and more improvements of the vehicle's components and active subsystems will influence the subjective driver feeling, as there are:

Component	influences:	implies :
• Tyre	Straight driving behaviour	Safety feeling
• Chassis	Frame stiffness	Good ground contact, riding comfort
• Servo steering	Steering feedback	Good ground contact
• Suspension control	Roll angle, static wheel travel	No change of payload

Hence, an electronic on-board payload monitoring system may be very helpful

1. as supportive driver information and
2. as additional input for any safety relevant active system(s).

3. IDENTIFICATION OF PAYLOAD

3.1 Levels of Payload Identification

In particular, vehicles with air spring suspension offer some appropriate possibilities to estimate the magnitude of the payload, as well as the position of its centre of gravity (CG) in a very accurate manner. In relation to the available vehicle configuration, three different levels of payload monitoring can be defined:

a) Axle load monitoring and longitudinal position of CG,

b) Wheel load monitoring and longitudinal and lateral position of CG,

c) Wheel load monitoring and full three-dimensional position of CG.

The following table focusses on these levels of payload monitoring systems.

Level	System requirements	Payload monitoring
a)	Simple air spring system for front, rear and trailer axles, semitrailer: only for tractor rear and trailer axles.	Static: Payload and longitudinal CG information and warnings while loading.
b)	Same as a), but independent left/right air spring system for rear axle(s) .	Static: Payload and 2-dim CG information and warnings while loading.
c)	Same as b)	Static: Same as b). Dynamic: Payload CG height.

Table 3.1: Basic scheme of payload monitoring

Typically of the payload identification, the highest level c) requires a dynamic solution in monitoring the payload height. Therefore, the identification process needs a definite, more or less long time period for the computation of the current CG height. This means, the driver will receive this information earliest *after* starting the drive. However, this should be sufficient in order to prevent roll over during the current transport.

The features of an air spring based payload identification system are shown and discussed in the following section.

3.2 Testing Results

The linearity of the relation between air spring pressure and the weighed axle load is shown in **figure 3.1** . The curves result from a static loading test on a tractor-semitrailer combination, where FA and RA denote the front and rear axle of the tractor, and TA denotes all the three axles of the trailer. The loading was done stepwise from empty to 14 test weights of 1.73 tons each, followed by stepwise unloading. Thus, the numbers given on the test weights denote the loading/unloading sequence. The diagram shows the quite good linearity of the pneumatic spring stiffnesses, which can advantageously be applied in the identification process. Furthermore, due to the air spring regulation system the hysteresis (caused by internal friction in the suspension system) is quite small.

The identification results of this loading test are shown in **figure 3.2** . As compared with the measured axle loads, the on-board identification provides quite accurate values within a range of 100 kg RMS. However, the possible deviations due to serial production have not been taken into consideration in the described basic results.

Next, the second level of payload monitoring is considered, which deals with the estimation of the wheel loads left/right in order to identify any lateral vehicle load. There is an important condition for solving this task: the vehicle must be equipped with an *independent* air spring system on the axle to be identified (that is mainly the vehicle's rear axle). In the following, some validations of a 19t MAN 4x2 truck are discussed.

When the load testings were performed, the test loads of 1 ton each were stepwise loaded accordingly to the figure, where the given numbers again denote the sequence of loading. The load is situated in a lateral right distance of 0.5 m off centre. **Figure 3.3** shows the air pressure - wheel load relation for this case of lateral load. In contrast to the central load, a remarkable hysteresis can be detected, caused by the angular distortion of the suspension system. However, this load/unload hysteresis can partially be compensated when using the air pressure *differences* in order to make an identification design. Furthermore, the overload of the right rear wheel is clearly seen on the diagram, where the axle reaches the bump stops.

The results of this test are shown in the **figures 3.4.** In spite of the above mentioned hysteresis, the axle load identification remains very accurate. Again the accuracy of the identification is within 1 percent of the payload weight, however, in the area of bumper contact (overloading) the estimation has failed. Anyway, the reach of maximum air spring pressure is a clear indicator for a warning signal against lateral overload.

The single wheel identification of the rear axle is done by an extended algorithm. Thus, the procedure is qualified to estimate the wheel load within a range of 3 percent of actual payload. The identification fails in the range of the bumper contact again.

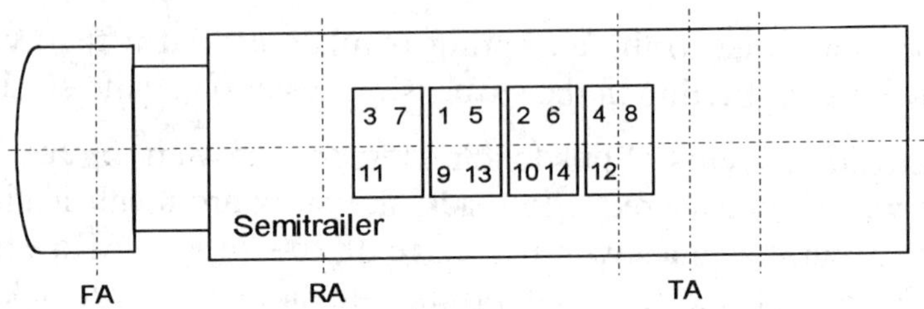

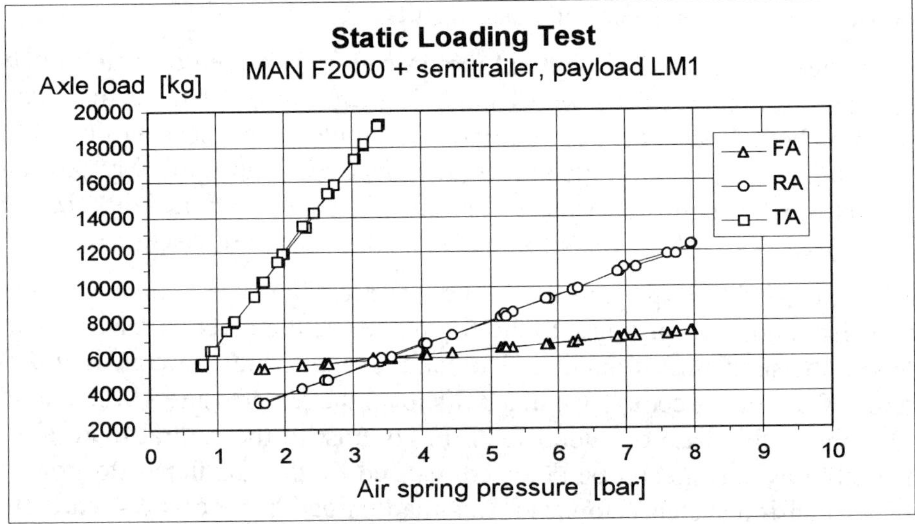

Figure 3.1: Pneumatic stiffness of the air springs

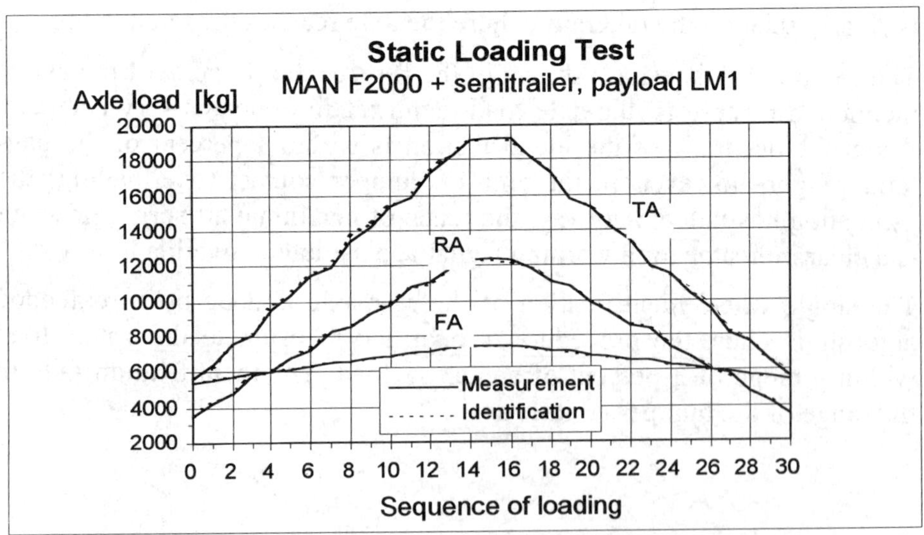

Figure 3.2: Comparison of axle loads: approach - measurement

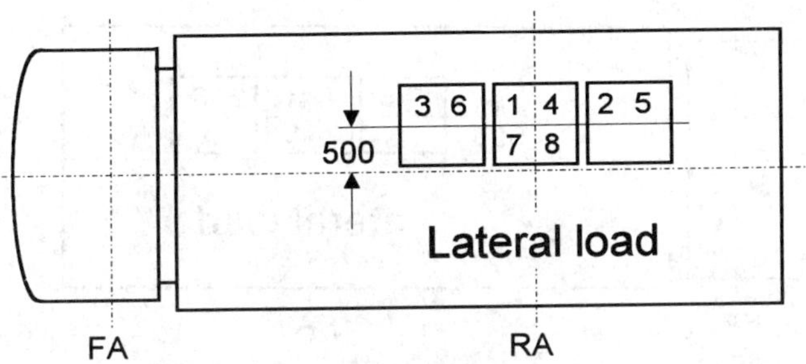

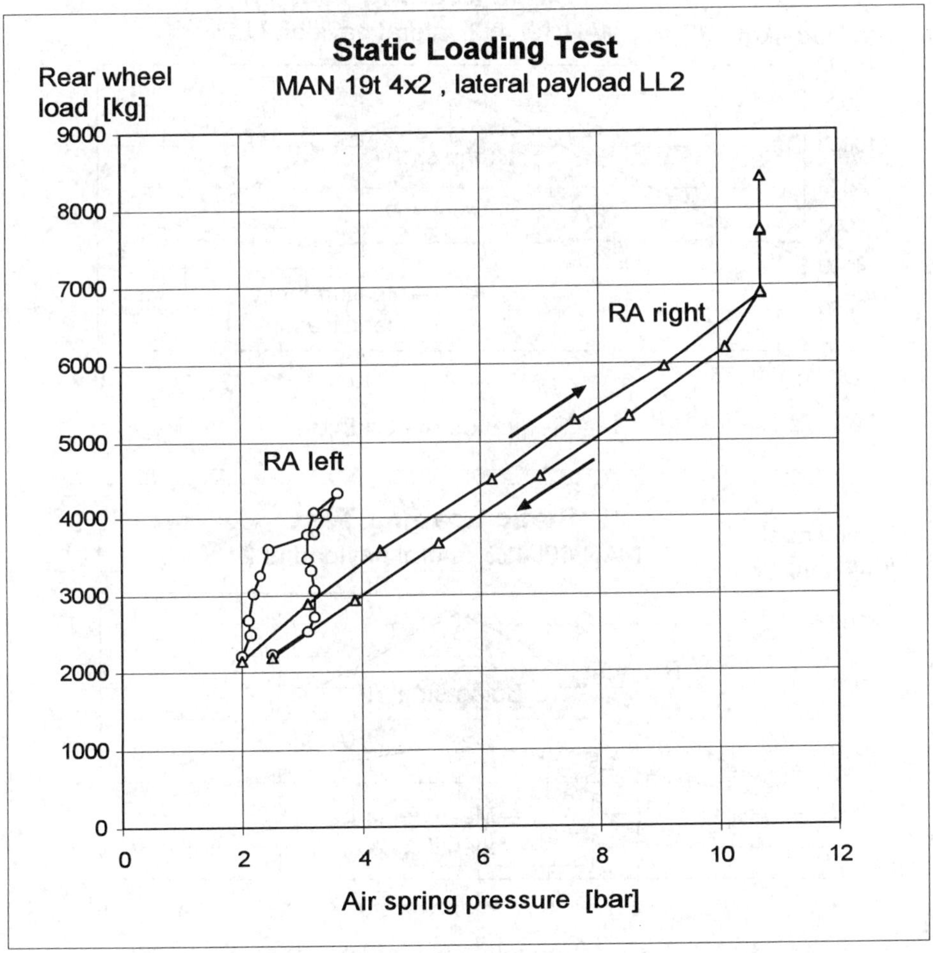

Figure 3.3: Pneumatic spring stiffness at lateral load

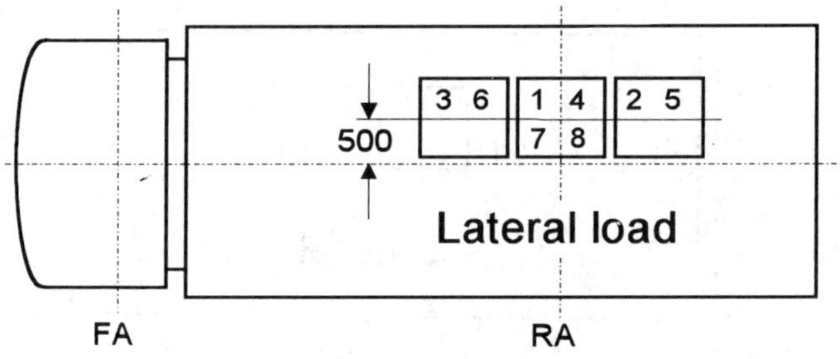

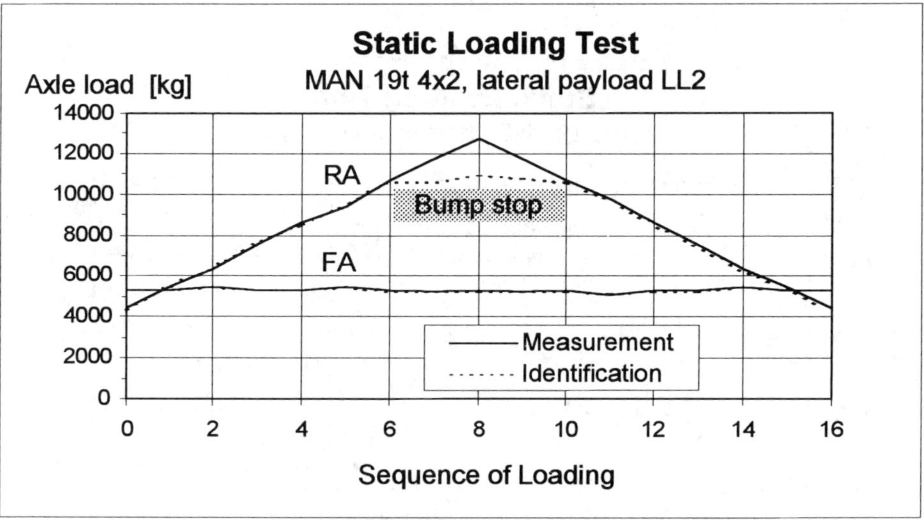

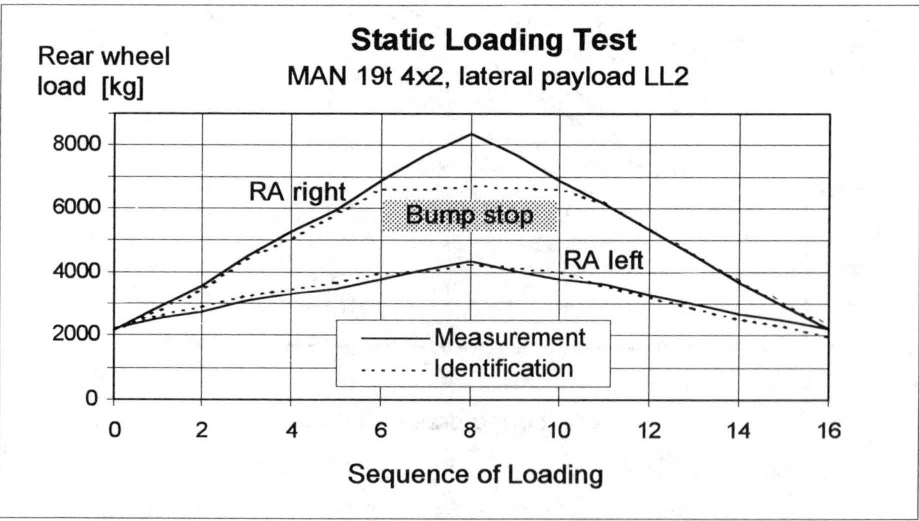

Figures 3.4: Comparison of axle/wheel loads: approach - measurement

Finally, the third level of payload identification - the detection of the load height - is described. As remarked above, this information is a very important one for a protective driver information as well as for an input quantity into safety relevant active subsystems.

The dynamic equilibrium between any applied roll torque and the torsional axle stabilization identifies the current state of the vehicle's roll motion. Therefore, the acting roll torque can be observed by the difference of the air spring pressures left/right. The disturbing rolling torque is caused by the product of load mass, its height above the roll centre and the lateral acceleration with respect to the load-fixed axis system. Hence, the rolling torque includes the disturbations due to the centripetal acceleration while cornering as well as the side inclinations of the road.

When using the air pressure differences for the observation of the acting rolling torque, there is one basic problem to be handled, see **figures 3.5** . The example shows the result from an accelerated/decelerated cornering test with a heavy 4x2 truck under full load. Due to the acting pneumatic stabilization control, the air pressure difference is continuously increasing while cornering. This control influence must be carefully compensated in order to perform a reliable identification of the payload height, see the second diagram. Thus, the constant value of payload height can be identified after a few seconds time of cornering.

Figure 3.6 shows a comparison of different load positions at the same test truck. The following three testing loads have been considered:

- Truck with empty cargo deck,
- Full load at the bottom of the cargo deck,
- Full load in high position.

First, the diagram shows a quite sufficient result of the payload identification process for the above mentioned variants. There remains a short period of convergence in the start up phase of cornering. Second, the typical behaviour of an experienced driver can be seen in the way he has been adjusting the lateral acceleration to the actual limits. Thus, the additional information about the magnitude of the load and its height may be a valuable support for the driver, either directly displayed or as input into any supportive active subsystem.

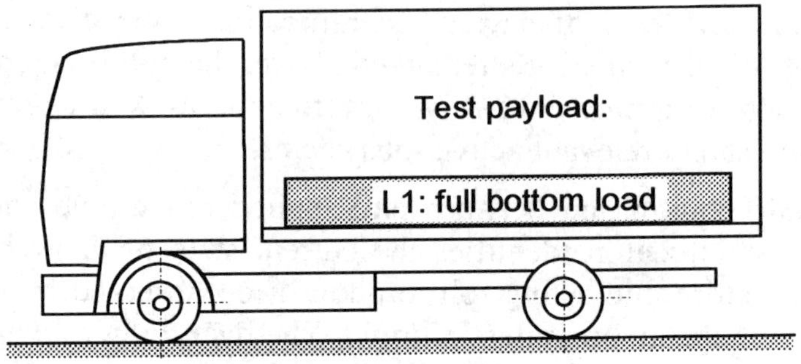

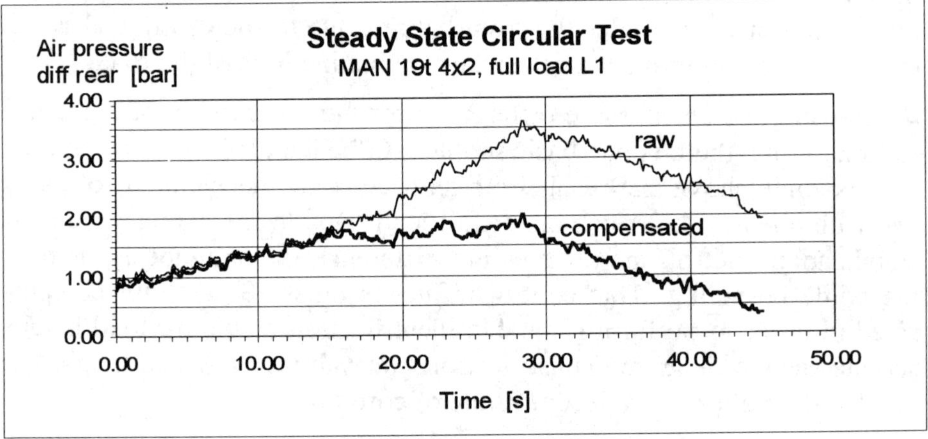

Figure 3.5 a: Compensation of roll stabilization control

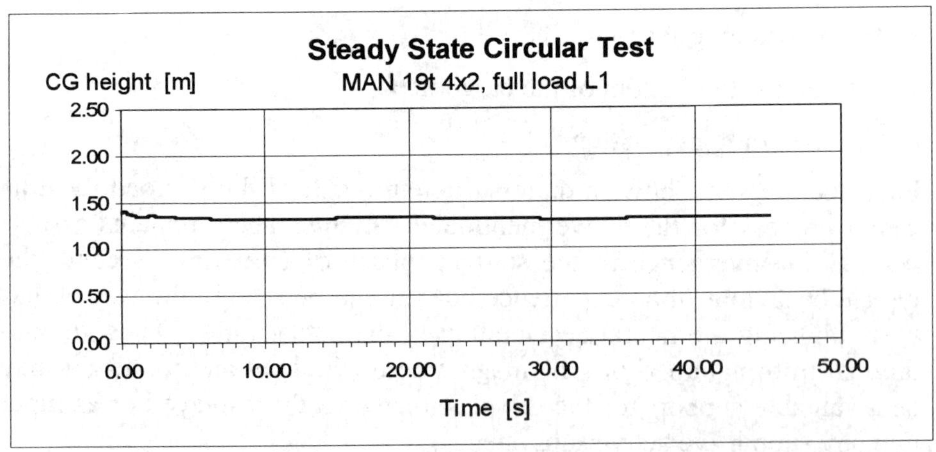

Figure 3.5 b: Identification of payload height

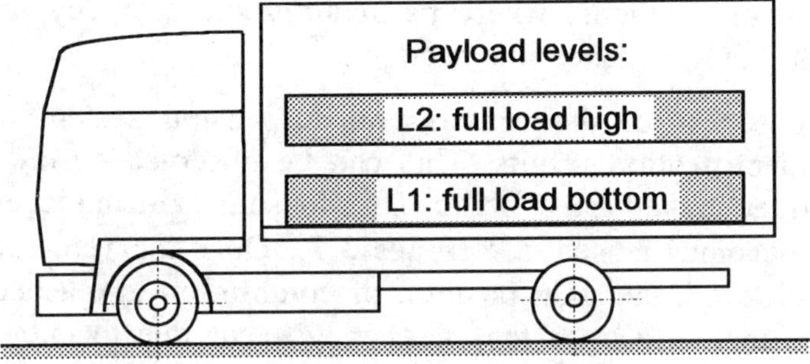

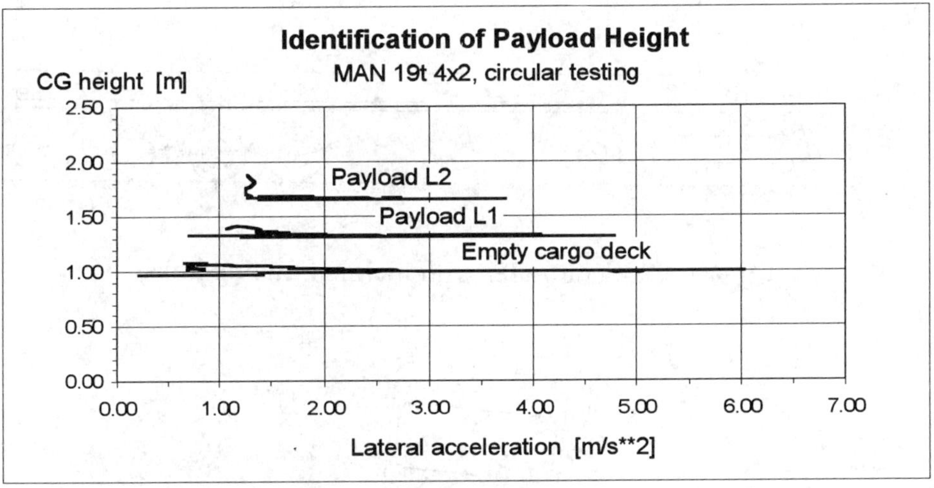

Figure 3.6: Identification of payload height

3.3 Remaining Problems

Even thought there are interesting ways for an effective and accurate monitoring of the current payload, some remaining problems have to be indicated. These problems, which are listed below, should be discussed with regard to appropriate solutions for the further serial application.

- Accurate payload and CG monitoring have had restricted to air sprung vehicles or vehicle-trailer combinations respectively. The corresponding monitoring systems for leaf sprung vehicles need total different identification methods, where particularly the accuracy and the robustness should be taken into account.

- Static tenseness of the chassis and suspension system may cause wrong identification results. This can be observed during loading a truck under locked hand brake. Due to some kinematic effects, the vehicle becomes tensed, see **figure 3.7** . Once the vehicle's brake is being unlocked, the right position of equilibrium is reached immediately. Further effects of tenseness may occur due to uneven stands, which cause internal distortions of the chassis frame (**figure 3.8**).

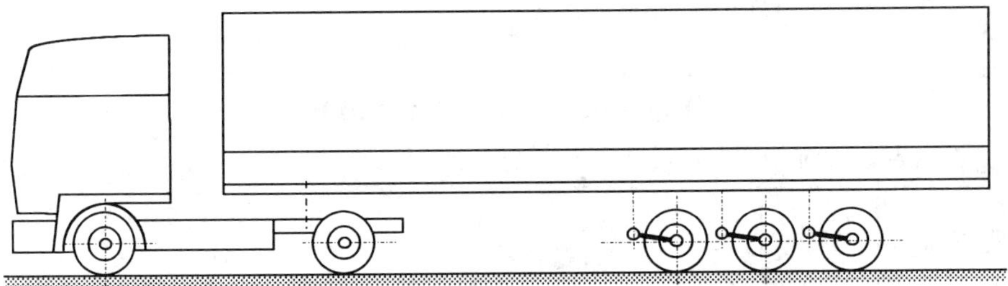

Figure 3.7: Semitrailer with inclined trailing links

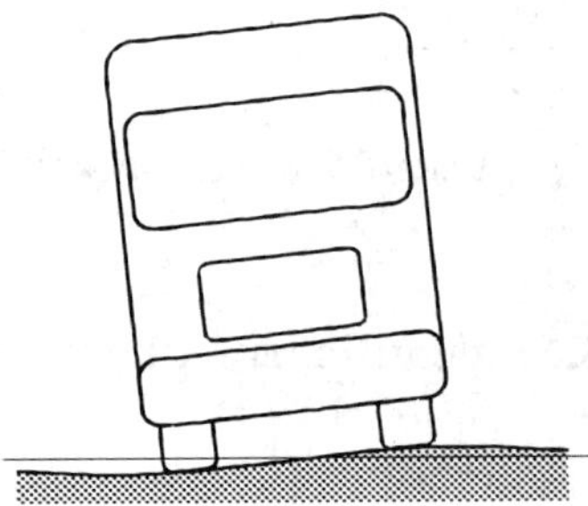

Figure 3.8: Truck distortion on uneven road surface

- The multitude of tractor - trailer/semitrailer combinations requires that each vehicle unit must *autonomously* identify and pass on its axle loads.

- Finally, it should be mentioned that the on-board identification of movable payloads (e.g. oscillating or fluid loads) has not fully been considered yet.

4. CONCLUSIONS

Due to the increasing motorization and the permanent improvements in chassis and suspension design of commercial vehicles, as well as the improved suspensions of the driver's cabins, the additional driver information concerning the actual loading state becomes relevant to an increasing degree. These information are particularly useful, if they are already available during the period of loading. Furthermore, additional information about the magnitude and the position of the payload during the transport can be used as input quantities into any safety relevant, electronic subsystem.

First, the present paper deals with some general aspects of the payload in commercial vehicles and its identification by the driver. In accordance to that, it focusses to different levels of supportive payload monitoring:

- Axle loads and longitudinal position of CG,

- Wheel loads and longitudinal and lateral position of CG,

- Wheel loads and full three-dimensional position of the payload.

Based on some recent testing results, the effectiveness and accuracy of the selected methods can be shown. However, there remain some problems which need further researches for getting solved. In particular, for the successful introduction of payload monitoring systems, it will be necessary to define the interfaces between both the autonomous systems at tractor and trailer.

5. REFERENCES

1. Jung C., Hirschberg W., Scheider F.: *Überwachung der Fahrsta bilität.* Technischer Schlußbericht der MAN Nutzfahrzeuge AG zum Forschungsvorhaben PROMETHEUS, München 1994.
2. Willumeit H.-P., Jürgenson T.: *Fahrermodelle - ein kritischer Überblick.* Automobiltechnische Zeitschrift Nr. 99 (1997).
3. Kusters L.: *Increasing roll-over Safety of Commercial Vehicles by Application of Electronic Systems*, Smart Vehicles, Swets & Zeitlinger, 1995
4. Jung C., Hirschberg W., Feigl E.: *Beladungserfassung von Nutzfahrzeugen*, Internal Reports, MAN Nutzfahrzeuge AG, 1996-1997

Monitoring and Assessment by Drivers with Special Needs, Simulator Experiences

Björn Peters

Drivers with special needs form a group of drivers who can not at all or only with serious problems manage to drive a standard production car. One reason for this is that ordinary cars are designed for people with full physical, mental and perceptual abilities. Another reason is that drivers with special needs have some form of impairment which limit their possibilities to cope with the technical environment they have to face in order to drive a car. The impairment also limits their overall independent mobility. Being able to drive a car is a way, perhaps the best way, for people with special needs to (re)gain mobility. Their chance to drive a car largely depends on the possibilities to adapt the car according to theirs abilities and resources. Unfortunately drivers with disabilities are rarely considered in the design of modern cars and new advanced driver support systems. This might decease their chances to drive but could also result in products that are far from what might be the best for all of us.

How many drivers with special needs are there? This is a difficult question to answer as it depends on who we consider being a driver with special needs. Usually we estimate that 10 - 15 % of the population have some kind of disability. Many of these are elderly. All types disabilities do not necessarily influence a persons ability to drive a car. For instance a hearing problem does not, at least legally, stop a person from driving. It has been estimated that 0.5% of European drivers are physically impaired and 0.2% cannot drive unless the car is adapted/converted. In Sweden there are between. 15.000 - 20.000 cars which are adapted for drivers with disabilities.

The focus in this presentation will be on drivers with upper and lower limb impairments and specially those with spinal cord injuries (SCI). These drivers constitute one of the larger subgroups of drivers with disabilities. This kind of impaired drivers were also the first to drive adapted cars. Disabled veterans, most with limb impairments, returning from the second world war were the first to express a significant demand for adapted cars. The adaptations most frequently needed are support systems for ingress and egress of the car and making controls possible to use with the limbs that are still working sufficiently. Most SCI drivers use their hands for all the primary control tasks (steering, braking and accelerating).

Are drivers with disabilities more accident prone? No, it looks at least like they drive just as safe as other drivers or even safer. They are not involved in more accidents and they seem to follow the same pattern as other drivers - elderly and novice drivers are more at risk. But this is an area that needs to be further investigated. On the one hand we know that these drivers have a different risk exposure as many of them restrict their driving by avoiding driving at rush hours, night time, bad weather etc. but also that they are closer to the limits of their resources once they drive. So you could say that they drive as safe as other drivers by voluntary restrictions and by spending a higher effort when driving. Discomfort is a limiting factor for their mobility. This could probably be improved as we monitor and assess their driving behaviour as a first step towards a new design.

Two simulator experiments have been performed in an advanced moving base driving simulator at the VTI with lower limb impaired drivers. The purpose of the first experiment was to 1. investigate if they drove different from a control group of matched non impaired drivers and 2. to identify possible problems they had while driving. Twenty-six tetraplegic drivers(lower and upper limb impaired, wheel chair users) and a control group of equal number drove a 80 km long country side route. The experimental group was divided into two equal subgroups who drove with two different types of hand controls for accelerating and braking. It turned out that the tetraplegic drivers drove just as well as the non impaired drivers except that they had a slightly longer but significant (5%) reaction time when they were presented to unexpected events. They also felt more tired from the driving task than the control group.

In the second experiment an Adaptive Cruise Control (ACC) system was installed in the driving simulator. Twenty drivers with lower limb impairment participated. All were experienced drivers of converted cars with hand controlled accelerator and brakes,. The purpose of this experiment was investigate how ACC driving would influence workload, comfort and driving behaviour. Two common types of hand controls were used (the same as in the first experiment). All subjects drove a 100 km long test route with oncoming traffic and car following situations both with and without ACC available. Subjective workload was found to be lower and performance better when ACC was used. The subjects thought they could control both speed and distance to leading vehicles better while driving with the ACC. The ACC system substantially contributed to decrease workload and increase comfort but need to be designed with respect to the demands and resources of this group of drivers.

Why should we bother with drivers with special needs? They are such a marginal group. There are at least two important reasons why they should not be neglected. First of all everybody should be provided with the best means to ensure sustained mobility. Public transportation facilities are not yet accessible in a way that it can compete with the independent mobility of driving a private car. This will surely also be profitable for the society. A second reason is that if we include these drivers in the design and evaluation process we stand a far better chance to early detect flaws in design and implementation of future cars and driver support systems. The ones with the least resources are more likely to early reveal the weak points in a car design, even those which might become a risk for the non impaired drivers in a critical situation.

1. IMPAIRMENT, DISABILITY, AND HANDICAP - WHAT IS THE DIFFERENCE?

Usually we don't bother to make any distinction between impairment, disability and handicap. In daily speech we call people who are deaf, blind, wheel-chair users and other impaired persons for handicapped people. But a handicap is not just an attribute linked to an individual but it also depends on how the environment is designed. *A handicap is caused by a mismatch between a disabled individual's needs and resources and the environment she or he has to interact with.* An impairment is a loss, abnormality, dysfunction in an individual's organ. A disability is a restriction or lack of ability in the activities an individual can perform compared to average human beings. A handicap is a disadvantage for an individual, caused by an impairment or a disability, that limits or prevents the fulfilment of a role that is normal for that individual. These terms have been defined and thoroughly explained by WHO [1]. Figure 1 shows that there are many people who are impaired but less who are disabled and even less that are handicapped. If the environment can be designed or adapted to users with impairments or disabilities they don't have to be handicapped or at least their handicap can be limited.

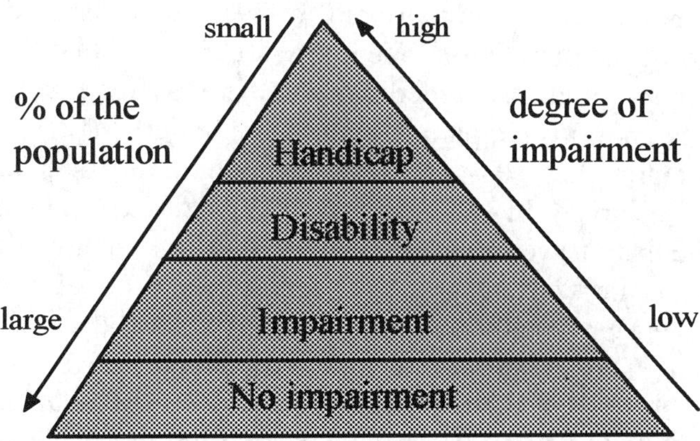

Figure 1 Impairment, disability, and handicap

Even though we make the distinction between these terms clear there is no clear cut way to decide when there is an impairment at hand or not. The levels are floating. When we consider car driving there are some medical requirements that have to be fulfilled in order to hold a driving licence. A hearing impairment does usually not a prevent a person from driving. Even deaf people are allowed to drive without any restrictions. But people with sight problems, or certain illness (epilepsy etc.), or balance problems are considered not able to drive. There are people with degraded performance that we normally does not normally consider being impaired. But where the reduced performance in one way or the other influence their chances to drive safe and comfortably. Many of these are elderly or senior citizens. These together with those who are disabled with respect to driving a standard production car we can say from a group of drivers that we call *drivers with special needs*.

2. HOW MANY ARE THERE?

As previously mentioned it is very difficult to clearly define the group of drivers with special needs. We can consider the figures for people with impairments and/or disabilities and then just note that the number of drivers with special needs will constitute in some cases an even larger group. Dependeing on the impairment. It seems that disabled people is a growing part of the population. We know for instance that the proportion of elderly people and also elderly drivers is steadily increasing. Many (70%) of the mobility impaired people are elderly ([2]). Sandhu and Woods [3] claim that 10 - 15 % of the population in most European countries are disabled. In 1988 Börjesson [2] estimated that approx. 12% of the Swedish travellers are disabled. How many drivers with disabilities are there? Haslegrave [4] tentatively estimated that 0.5% of the drivers were physically impaired and 0.2% needed an adapted car in order to drive. This meant at that time over 70,000 driver under 65 year in England. In Sweden there are between 15 - 20.000 adapted cars. This implies that 0.3 - 0.4 % of the driving population in Sweden use adapted cars. This is a slightly higher proportion than what Haslegrave reported. This could be due to a better financial situation for drivers with disabilities in Sweden than in England. Divers with limb (upper and/or lower) impairments is quite a large group people who require adapted cars. Drivers with spinal cord injuries constitute a rather small part of the drivers but they are a group of drivers with whom much of the adaptation experience have been gained. If we consider drivers with special needs that would benefit from an adapted or rather an improved design of the driver's cab we'll end up with quite a large part of the driving population.

3. SPINAL CORD INJURIES AND DRIVING

A *spinal cord injury* (SCI) means that both the sensory and motor nerve function is impaired. A SCI is caused by a disconnection in the spinal nerves. These nerves are vital for our ability to move. A dysfunction in the spinal nerves can have many causes but I will here only discuss traumatic SCI. This kind of damage will make an individual more or less paralysed in the limbs. But other functions in the nervous system will be intact like perceptual, cognitive, memory abilities.

The spine is divided in to 5 section (cranial, thoracic, lumbar, sacral and caudal). Nerves that control different parts of the body enter the spine at different levels. Figure 2 gives a picture of how the nerves are distributed along the body. The location of a spinal injury determines the extent of the paralysis. The part of the body that is below the injury will be affected. An injury located to the torso (T 1 - T12) will result in a lower limb impairment (*paraplegi*) and if the injury is located to the neck (C1 - C8) will also affect the upper limb (*tetraplegi*). If an lesion is located at C4 or above the person will not be able to drive.

SCI is a typical injury for young males. Over the years the gender distribution have been 80% males and 20% females and the mean age when injured somewhere between 20 and 30. Now though it seems like the ladies are catching up (30 - 35%) and also we can see an increase in age (35 - 40) at the time of injury. A largest part of these injuries are caused by traffic accidents but it has decreased lately ([5]).

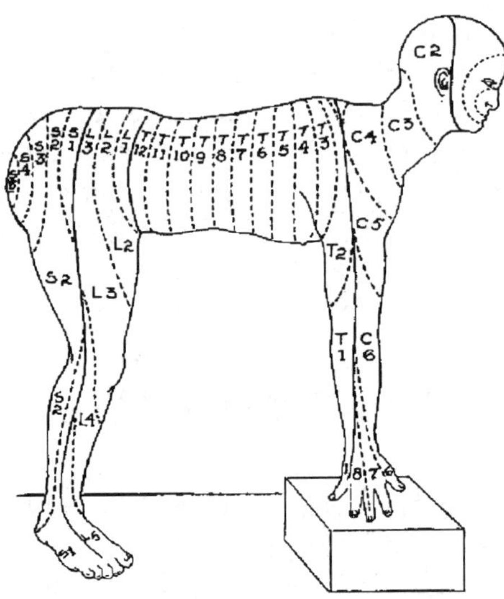

Figure 2 The distribution of the nerves that control different parts of the body with respect to where they enter the spinal cord (C = cranial, T = thoracic L = lumbar, S = sacral)

SCI will greatly reduce the mobility and independence for the individual affected. Many will need a wheel chair for their personal mobility. A paraplegic will be able to use a manual wheel chair but tetraplegics with a lesion located at a high level will probably need an electric wheel chair. Driving an adapted car will be the best way to regain mobility and independence for those who can. Public transport and special transport services cannot at yet offer the same level of independent mobility.

A person with a disability who wants to drive will be assessed in order to find out if the reduced abilities are not too extensive and if the available resources will be enough in order to drive an adapted car. The basic requirement is that the car should be adapted in order to permit the disabled person to drive just as safe as all other drivers. Apart from the medical assessment a dedicated driver assessment is usually performed which include *reaction time test, reach, force, endurance* etc. Some times the assessment also includes perceptual and cognitive tests but this is not usually the case at least for persons with SCI. Preferably the assessment should also include some kind of initial driving test. This is a procedure applied in many assessment centres in England like at Banstead Mobility Centre [6]. In the US they have also developed a instrumented test vehicle especially designed for SCI driver applicants

[7]. How driving simulator can be used to assess drivers with disabilities have been described by Verwey [8]. All these assessments can also serve a more general purpose; namely to let us better understand what human resources are needed in order to drive a car.

The most common adaptations for SCI drivers are support systems for entering and leaving the car, adapted primary and secondary controls. Here the focus will be on adapted primary controls. Most SCI drivers cannot use their feet for the pedals and they have to use hand controls for the accelerator and the brake [9]. Even if the car is adapted it is known that many impaired drivers and not the least the SCI drivers suffer from physical overload caused by the driving task [10].

4. ACCIDENTS AND INCIDENTS

It could be expected that drivers who need to spend more effort and work closer to the limit of their abilities in order to drive would be more accident prone. But it does not seem to be so. Or at least as far as we know now. First of all we have to note that our knowledge about the accidents and incidents of disabled drivers is both incomplete and unclear [11], [4]. But there are some investigations which show that these drivers are involved in accidents to the same or even lower extent as other drivers and that they show the same accident pattern which means that elderly and inexperienced drivers are more involved in accidents [12], [13]. Lääperi et al. found in a retrospective study with a group of 105 drivers who had various disabilities that 7.6 % had been involved in an accident which is slightly higher than for the total population (7.0%). But when they also consider the exposure (yearly driven distance) they found that the result was reversed 3.8% per 10^6 km for the drivers with disabilities compared to 4.0 % per 10^6 km for all. The largest group of drivers that Lääperi studied had SCI (60%). We can conclude that there is no obvious evidence that SCI drivers should be more at risk compared to the total driving population. But there is a great need for further studies in this area. At least we know that the passive safety in converted cars is not what is ought to be but and that the active safety, usefulness, and comfort of adapted primary controls needs to be further studied and developed [14].

5. DRIVING SIMULATOR EXPERIMENTS WITH SCI DRIVERS

The dynamic driving simulator at the VTI was used in both the experiments described below. The car body used in the simulator was the front half of a Saab 9000 with an automatic gearbox. The vehicle dynamics is modelled in the computer system and the moving base system simulates accelerations in three directions through roll, pitch and linear lateral motions. The visual system presents the external scenario on a 120° wide screen, 2.5 metres in front of the driver. The sound system generates noise and infrasounds that resembles the internal environment in a driving car. The vibration system simulates the

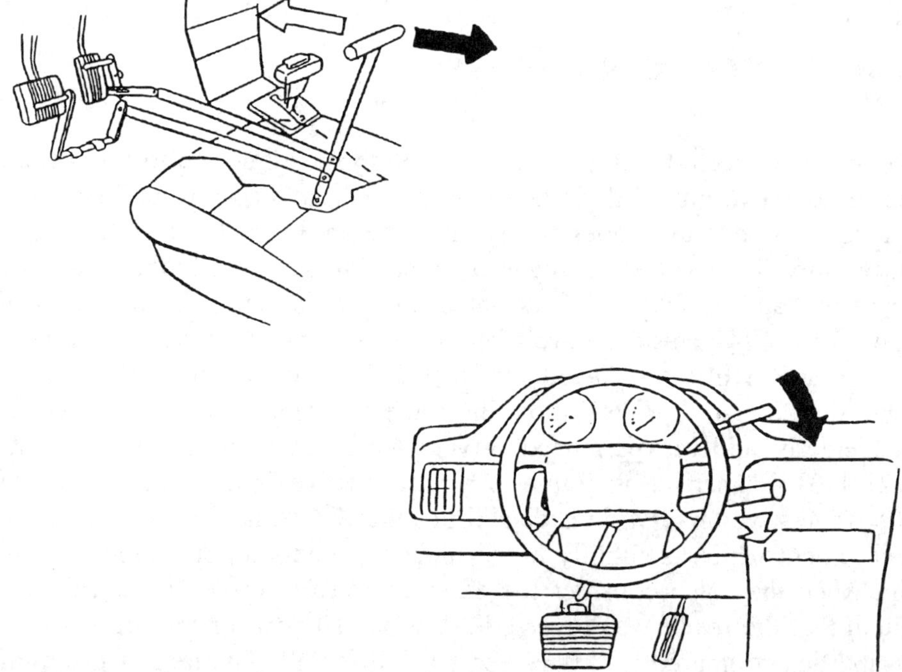

Figure 3 Hand controls for accelerator and brake. To the left is a single lever system and to the right is a dual lever system, separate levers for acceleration and braking. The white arrows show the direction of operation for braking and the black arrow indicates how the accelerator lever work. (from SINTEF, Unimed, Norway)

sensations the driver experience from the contact between the road and the vehicle. The driving simulator have high performance characteristics with very short time delay of maximum 40 ms. A short time delay between visual and motion perception is important to prevent motion sickness and to maintain a high level of reality. The car body is positioned 2 metres above floor level. To make it accessible for the SCI subjects, a wheel chair lift was installed and the platform outside the car body was extended. No other adaptations were done for entering and leaving the car.

Two common systems for hand controlled accelerator and brakes were installed in the simulator (Figure 3). The single lever system was operated by the driver so that he or she pushed the lever forward for braking and pulled it to accelerate. The other system had two separate levers placed on the steering column. The brake lever was pushed, and the accelerator lever was moved radially. Both systems were operated by the driver's right hand. The left hand was used for steering.

6. DRIVING BEHAVIOUR OF TETRAPLEGIC DRIVERS

The objective with the first experiment was to investigate driving behaviour of two groups of SCI drivers as compared to non disabled drivers[15]. Fifty-two subjects, 26 SCI (tetraplegi) drivers and 26 able-bodied persons, participated in the study. The SCI drivers were paralysed in their lower limbs, impaired the upper limbs and had trunk instability problems all due to an spinal cord lesion at neck level (C4-C7). They all depended on a wheel chair for their personal mobility. The gender distribution for both groups were 24 males and 2 females. The subjects were divided in to two subgroups equal in size depending on the type of hand control (single or dual lever system) they used in the simulator. All SCI drivers were experienced drivers with their respective hand controls for accelerator and brake. The control group consisted of 26 able-bodied subjects and was matched to the experimental group concerning gender, age, driving experience, and annual distance driven. The control subjects used the car's original pedals for braking and accelerating.

The subjects drove on a two-lane, 9 m wide asphalt road with high friction. The weather condition was slightly cloudy with a sight distance of approximately 400 m. The test route was 80 km long and consisted of a mixture of straight and curve sections with various radius. It resembled an ordinary rural road. There were oncoming traffic and parked cars that the driver had to pass along the route. To simulate unexpected traffic events requiring the driver to react, a visual stimulus (red or yellow square) was presented on the screen, peripherally in the visual field on the left side of the road. The subjects' task was to brake as fast as possible when red squares were presented (4 times), and to do nothing when yellow squares were presented (4 times). All subjects drove the same route and were exposed to the same situations and events.

Subjects were give verbal and written instructions before the test. They also drove a 20 km route before the actual test in order to familiarise them with the driving simulator. After the test they rated their workload and answered a questionnaire.

The mean speed and lateral position over the total test route (80 km) was calculated for each subject, and group means were created. The mean speed for the SCI drivers was 91.3 km/h, while the controls drove with an average speed of 88.4 km/h. There were no significant (5%) differences between the SCI drivers and the control group with respect to speed and lateral position. Also there were no differences between the two subgroups of SCI driver in this respect. The mean variation in lateral position was calculated over all *straight* sections for each subject. There was no significant (5%) difference between the SCI group (SD=.43 m) and the control group (SD=.47 m). But for the two experimental subgroups there was a difference [F(1,24)=5.30, p=.0303]. The subjects driving with the dual lever system had a greater variation in lateral position (SD=.47 m) compared to those driving with the single lever system (SD=.40 m). The mean reaction time for the group of SCI drivers was 0.90 s and for the control group 0.80 s. This difference was significant [F(1,50)=6.53, p=.0137. The two subgroups of SCI drivers did not differ significantly (5%). The six workload factors of NASA-TLX were analysed and the only significant difference between the tetraplegic and control groups was found for time pressure [F(1,50=8.42, p=.0055]. The tetraplegics experienced a heavier time pressure compared to the controls. All subjects had to answer the question "Do you think it was tiring to brake and accelerate?" and the answers were given on a rating scale ranging from 1 for "very tiring" to 7 for "not at all tiring". A one-way ANOVA showed a significant [F(1,50)=9.65, p=.00312] difference between the SCI group (5.77) and the control group (6.81). The tetraplegic subjects thought it was physically more tiring to brake and accelerate compared to the able-bodied subjects. The tetraplegic drivers using the single lever hand control thought it was physically more tiring to brake and accelerate (5.08) compared to the tetraplegic drivers using the dual lever hand control (6.46). Static force was measured before and after the test but did not reveal any difference between the various groups.

It was concluded that compared to non impaired drivers using conventional pedals, SCI drivers driving with hand controlled brake and accelerator

- show the same overall driving behaviour.
- react somewhat slower to unexpected traffic events.
- do not rate their workload level higher.
- but feel more tired from braking and accelerating, an experience which can not be explained by physical local fatigue.

If the two subgroups of SCI driver are considered separately

- the drivers using the dual lever control have a greater variation in lateral position (swerve)
- the drivers using the single lever control feel more tired from braking and accelerating.

7. DRIVERS WITH LOWER LIMB IMPAIRMENTS DRIVING WITH AN ADAPTIVE CRUISE CONTROL

The purpose of the study was to investigate ACC driving influence on workload, comfort and driving behaviour compared to manual driving[16]. The ACC system used in this experiment could keep a constant speed selected and set by the driver and also adapt speed in order to keep a safe distance to a leading vehicle.

Twenty SCI subjects, seventeen men and three women, participated in this study. All subjects were experienced drivers of adapted cars. The subjects were divided in to two subgroups equal in size depending on the type of hand control (single or dual lever system) they used for manual driving. The same types of hand controls as in the previously described was used also in this experiment. The rather few number of female subjects (15%) corresponds to the gender distribution among lower limb disabled people in general. All subjects had a minimum driving experience of at least 2 years (mean 9.7 years) or at least 40,000 km in adapted cars equipped with the type of hand control they used in this study. All subjects drove both with and without the ACC available.

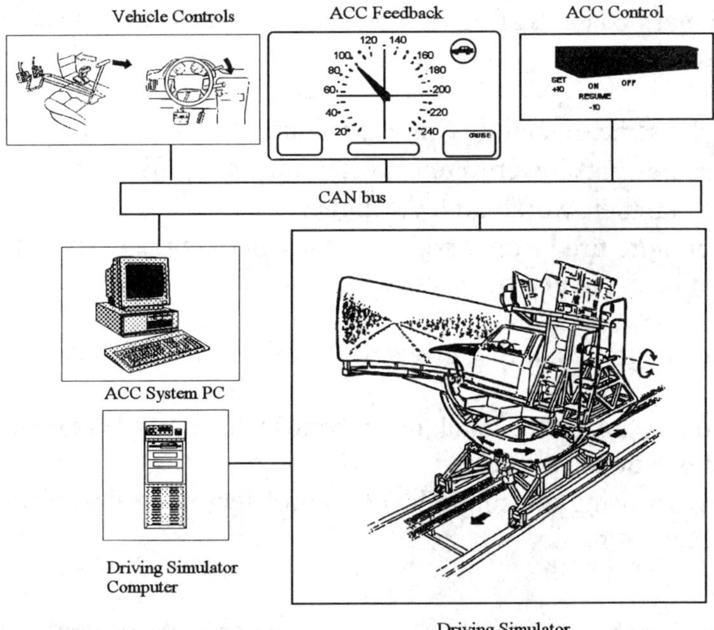

Figure 4 Simulator set-up for the ACC experiment

The ACC system was installed in the driving simulator. All communication between the ACC and the driving simulator was handled by a CAN bus (Figure 4). Basically the ACC worked as a standard CC by keeping a set cruising speed selected by the driver, but it could also adjust speed in order to maintain a safe distance to a leading vehicle. This function was realised by a simulated sensor for vehicle detection mounted in the front of the car. The ACC controlled both throttle and brakes when activated. The selected speed could be adjusted up and down in increments of 10 km/h by the driver. Speeding overrode the ACC, but the selected speed was resumed when the accelerator was released. The driver could at any time disengage the ACC by braking or turning the ACC off manually. After braking the ACC could resumed previous speed if the speed was not below 30 km/h. Headway applied by the ACC was speed dependent. Feedback to was provided on the dash-board. When the ACC was turned on the word CRUISE would appear in amber at the lower right on the dash-board. The speedometer had a circle of amber which indicated selected speed. At the top right on the dash board an amber car symbol was lit when a leading vehicle was identified. The ACC controls were placed on the direction indicator stalk to the left of the steering column. The controls had the following functions ON/OFF, SET/RESUME, Step Up (+ 10 km/h) and Step Down (- 10 km/h).

The test road was 9 m wide with two lanes and a hard shoulder. The road surface consisted of asphalt with randomised texture with high friction. It was daylight conditions with a sight distance of approximately 500 m. The route consisted of mixed straight sections and sections with varying horizontal and vertical curvature. The speed limit, marked by road signs, was in general 90 km/h but occationally also 70 km/h. The experimental route was 100 km long. The same route was used for all subjects and both with and without ACC.

Different traffic situations appeared in a randomised sequence but equal to all subjects during the driving session. The subjects were meeting oncoming vehicles. Unexpected traffic events were simulated by visual stimulus as for the previously described experiment. There were sixteen car following situations during the test drive. Catching up procedure was standardised. There were four types of car following situations: Leading vehicle braking, Leading vehicle driving with varying speed, Leading vehicle with constant speed, Leading vehicle stopping at traffic lights.

The following *measures* were used: speed, lateral position on the road, time headway, and reaction time. Subjective measures of workload (NASA - RTLX) and questionnaires were used to collect the subject's opinion. Before the test all subjects were give written and verbal instructions and answered a questionnaire about age, gender, handicap, and driving experience. All subjects were instructed to drive and interact with other road users as they would do normally in real life traffic under comparable conditions. At both occasions, with and without ACC, the subjects drove a 20 km long training route where all the relevant traffic situations were demonstrated. After the test drive all subjects rated the experienced workload and in a separate questionnaire answered questions regarding speed and distance control, and usability of the ACC system.

The *general driving behaviour* was analysed in terms of mean speed and lateral position on the road and the variations of these measures. The mean speed level was for ACC driving 88.6 km/h (single lever drivers 89.3 km/h and dual lever drivers 87.8 km/h) and for No ACC driving 89.1 km/h (single lever drivers 88.2 km/h and dual lever drivers 89.9 km/h). A two-way ANOVA did not show any significant (5%) interactions or main effects.

Free flow driving was defined as the total distance when the subjects did not have to deal with catching up, overtaking, or other interfering situations. The total free flow driving distance was approximately 60 km (60%) of the total route. The *mean speed* for free flow driving was for the ACC condition 94.7 km/h (single lever drivers 95.4 km/h and dual lever drivers 94.1 km/h) and for No ACC driving 96.3 km/h (single lever drivers 95.0 km/h and dual lever drivers 97.6 km/h). There were no main or interaction effects (5%). The variation in speed (Figure 5) was for the ACC condition 3.3 km/h (equal for both groups) and for No ACC driving 4.7 km/h (single lever drivers 5.3 km/h and dual lever drivers 4.1 km/h). The difference between ACC and No ACC was significant ($F(1,36) = 6.59$, p= .0145).

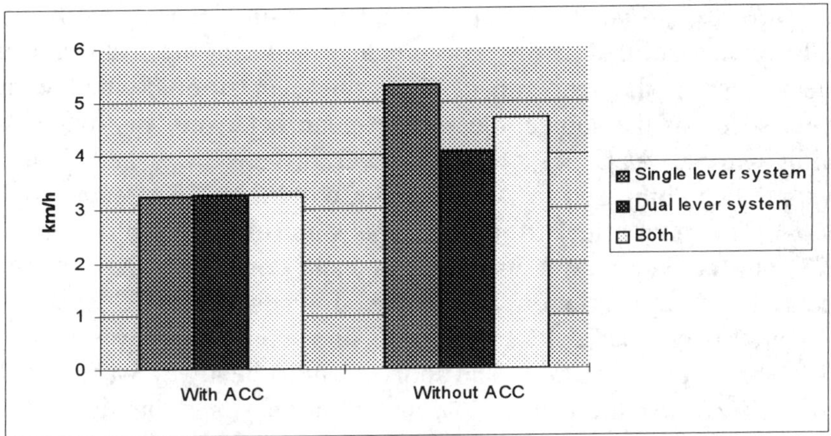

Figure 5 Variation in speed with and without ACC available

Manual speed keeping imposes a constant load on the driver. Variation in speed (km/h) during free flow driving was analysed to detect possible degradation in manual speed keeping compared to ACC driving. The difference increased with distance driven (Figure 6)

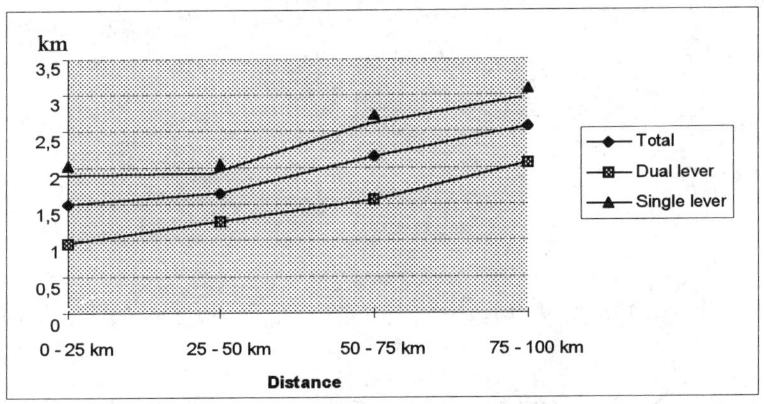

Figure 6 Difference in speed variation (km) between No ACC and ACC condition

Mean (n = 4) reaction time for red squares were calculated for all subjects. The mean reaction time for the ACC condition was 1.32 s (1.41 s for single lever drivers and 1.23 s for dual lever drivers) and 1.43 s for the No ACC condition (1.50 s for single lever drivers and 1.37 s for dual lever drivers). There were no interaction or main effects (5%).

Car following situations were analysed with respect to headway. Headway was defined as the time distance between the front end of the subject's car to the rear end of the vehicle in front divided with the current speed of the subject's car. The mean headway was longer while driving without ACC 3.3 s (single lever drivers 3.2 s and dual lever drivers 3.4 s) compared to ACC driving condition 2.6 s (same for both groups). The main effect from ACC was significant ($F(1,36) = 8.82$, $p = .0053$) but there was no main effect of hand control nor any interaction effects. Headway variation was reduced when the ACC system was available 1.0 compared to 1.4 s. Also this main effect was significant ($F(1,36) = 15.68$, $p = .003$). The shortest (min) headway was considered to be critical for the car following situations. The number of short headway deceased while driving with the ACC (figure 7). Without ACC 50% were equal or below 1 s and with ACC this was reduced to 20%.

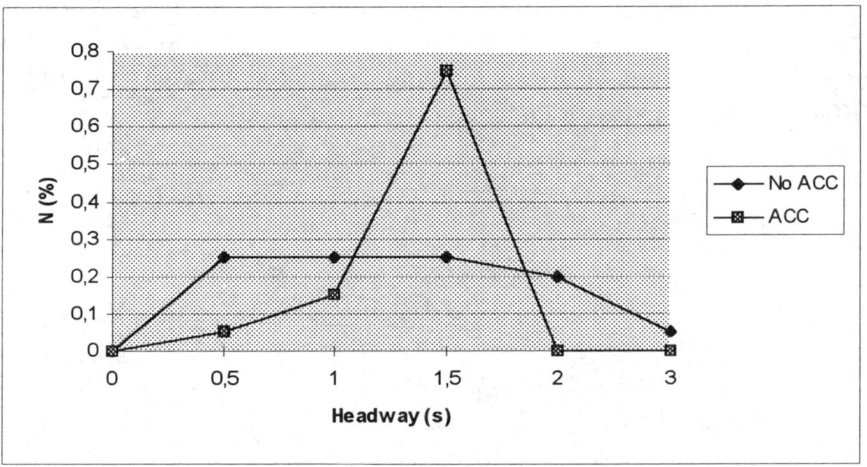

Figure 7 Distribution of min headway during 14 car following situations

NASA - RTLX was used to assess workload. Each subject rated the six workload factors; *mental demand, physical demand, time pressure, performance, effort, and frustration level* on separate continuous scales ranging from very low (0) to very high (100). The total driving task was rated as more loading with No ACC than with ACC (Figure 8). Two-way ANOVAs revealed significant main effects of ACC mode for four factors: physical demand ($F(1,36) = 10.13$; $p = .0030$), time pressure ($F(1,36) = 6.13$; $p = .0181$), performance ($F(1,36) = 4.12$; $p = .0497$), and effort ($F(1,36) = 4.67$; $p = .0373$). No main effects of hand control or interaction effects were found.

The subjects were asked to rate how well they could control speed level and how much effort they had to assign to control it. The same types of questions were asked for the distance control to a vehicle ahead. Scales with seven steps were used ("1" = very bad / no effort and "7" = very well / very high effort). Both groups rated the control to be higher and effort to be lower for the ACC condition: speed keeping (ACC mean = 6.2, No ACC mean = 4.0), speed keeping effort (ACC mean = 1.6, No ACC mean = 3.6), distance keeping (ACC mean = 5.8, No ACC mean = 4.6), distance keeping effort (ACC mean = 1.7, No ACC mean = 3.0). All differences were significant ($p < 0.015$) but there were no main effects of type of hand control and no interaction effects (figure 9).

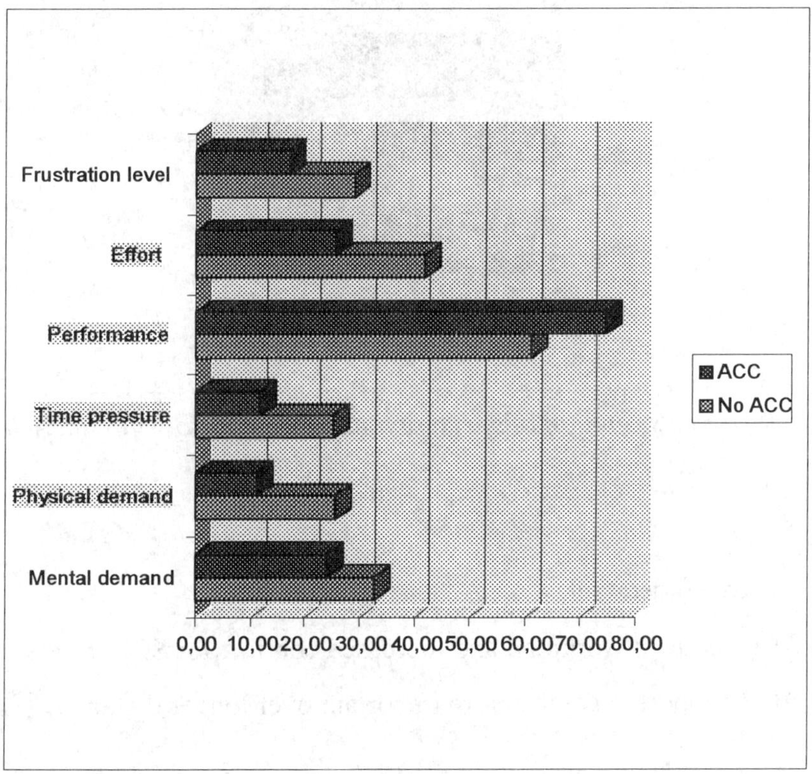

Figure 8 Mean workload ratings for both groups (n=20) with and without ACC.

The subjects were also asked rate some aspects considered to be important for ACC usage and acceptance. A seven point rating scale was used. The results were "General opinion of the ACC?" (mean = 6.7 sd = 0.75), "ACC contribution to comfort?" (mean = 6.5 sd = 0.95), "Learn to use ACC?" (mean = 6.7 sd = 0.59), "Trusting ACC?" (mean = 6.5 sd = 0.69), "Wanting to have ACC?" (mean = 6.9 sd = 0.45), "ACC better than own CC?" (mean = 6.5 sd = 0.77). Even though the ACC was well received the subjects pointed out that the ACC controls were not optimal with respect to their needs and resources.

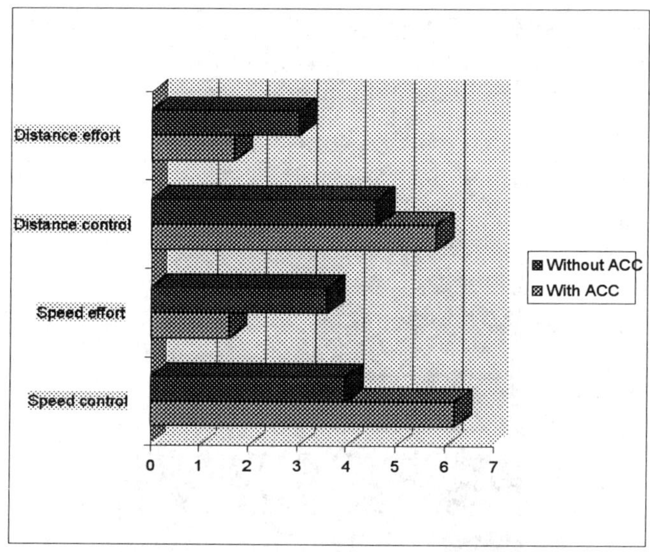

Figure 9 Driver's opinion of speed and distance control with and without ACC

It was concluded that:

* ACC reduced workload and increased comfort for SCI drivers

* ACC support becomes more important over longer distances

* ACC was rated to improve speed and distance control in car following situations

* ACC system was well accepted, wanted and trusted

* ACC driving produced a shorter mean time headways compared to manual driving

* ACC had no effects on speed level, variation in lateral position, or reaction time.

* ACC driving did not influence workload, comfort, and driving behaviour differently with respect to type of hand control used

8. WHY SHOULD WE CONSIDER DRIVERS WITH SPECIAL NEEDS?

Even if the two experiments described here did not reveal any great design flaws it is obvious that the potential users with the least resources will determine the overall usefulness of a system. Including drivers with special needs will most likely enhance the market potential for new cars and in-car support systems. This becomes even more pronounced when we consider that the proportion of elderly drivers will steadily increase during the forth coming decades. Driving simulators are certainly not the only way to study and assess driver behaviour and it should not be viewed as an alternative to field trials and other tests but as a complement. We need all of it. And we need both qualitative and quantitative assessment methods. A driving simulator have some important advantages like a completely controlled environment, a possibility to study safety critical situations without any risk to the driver and in a simulator it is fairly simple to test new systems at an early stage of development. But the simulator has to put driver in such a situation that feels like real driving. The experiments described did not really include any safety critical situations. And safety is of course a crucial aspect of adapted cars but there are also other aspects that need to be considered like: Can the driver use the converted controls?, Does the controls function the way the user believes and expects? Does the driver get adequate feedback. Is it comfortable to use? What happens when there is a malfunction in the system? What happens when the car is crashed? There are many questions that needs to be answered before the car is adapted to the needs and resources of drivers with special needs. We certainly need to further develop the assessment methods for drivers with special needs. Assessing drivers with special needs will serve at least two purposes: 1. A way to provide better car adaptations and 2. A possibility understand what resources are needed to drive a car. Preferably cars should be designed in a way that the needs for adapting it should be minimal. Designing a car that suits all that can drive is probably not feasible but if we try to eliminate the most serious obstacles and not introduce more we will probably get better cars for all. A design for all.

REFERENCES

1. WHO, *International Classification of Impairments, Disabilities, and Handicaps*, . 1980, WHO: Geneva.
2. Börjesson, M., *Kollektivtrafik för alla. Sammanfattning av resultat från TFB-stödd forskning och utveckling om handikappade och trafik*, . 1988, TFB: Stockholm.
3. Sandhu, J.S. and T. Wood, *Demography and market sector analysis of people with special needs in thirteen European countries: A report on Telecommunication Usability Issues*, . 1990, Newcastle Polytechnic: Newcastle upon Tyne.
4. Haslegrave, C.M., *Driving for Handicapped People*, in *Ergonomics in Rehabilitation*, A. Mital and W. Karwowski, Editors. 1988, Taylor & Francis: Philadelphia. p. 13 - 34.
5. Kreuter, M., *Ryggmärgsskador - orsaker, köns och åldersfördelning (SCI - causes, gender and age dsitribution)*,, personal communication. 1997.
6. Banstead_Mobility_Centre, *Annual Report*, . 1996, Banstead Mobility Centre: Carshalton, Surrey.
7. Hicks, G.W., *Anatomy of an Instrumented Generic Quadriplegic Evaluation Van*, . 1993, SAE: Warrendale.
8. Verwey, W.B., *On Evaluating Vehicle Adaptations for Disabled Drivers*, . 1994, TNO Institute for Perception: Soesterberg, Holland.
9. Naniopoulos, A. and E.B. (eds.), *Existing aids for DSN (Drivers with Special Needs*, . 1992, University of Thessaloniki: Thessaloniki, Greece.
10. Nicolle, C., B. Peters, and P.H. Vossen. *Towards the Development of ATT Guidelines for Drivers with Special Needs*. in *First World Congress on Applications of Transport Telematics and Intelligent Vehicle-Highway Systems*. 1994. Paris, France: Artech House, London.
11. Transportforskningsdelegationen, *Handikappade fordonsförares säkerhet Kunskapsöversikt*, . 1980, Transportforskningsdelegationen - tfd: Stockholm.
12. Simms, B. and L. O'Toole, *Driving assessment of disabled people 1988 - 1990*, . 1993, TRL: Crowthorne.

13.   Lääperi, T., *et al. Traffic accident risk of disabled drivers having special driving control equipment: A driver survey and accident data.* in *Scandinavian Medical Society of Paraplegia (SMSOP).* 1995. Oslo, Norway.

14.   Koppa, R.J., *State of the Art in Automotive Adaptive Equipment.* Human Factors, 1990. **32**(4): p. 439 - 456.

15.   Peters, B. and L. Nilsson. *Driving Performance of DSN (Drivers with Special Needs) using Hand Controls for Braking and Accelerating.* in *26th International Symposium on Automotive Technology and Automation (ISATA).* 1993. Aachen, Germany: Automotive Automation Ltd, London.

16.   Peters, B. *Evaluation of an Adaptive Cruise Control (ACC) System used by Drivers with Lower Limb Impairments.* in *Thrid World Congress on Intelligent Transport Systems.* 1996. Orlando, USA.

Vehicle Performance: J.P. Pauwelussen (ed.) pp. 46-66

Vehicle Handling Aspects for Drivers with Special Needs

Aleid Hekstra and Rinus Kempeneers

The requirements and assessment criteria to determine the medical fitness to drive and the driving skills of the European driver are outlined in the driving licence directive (91/439/EEG). All drivers must comply to these criteria. An expert judgement on compliance is made at least once for each driver before the issuing of the driving licence. These requirements are not based on physical measures in relation to the vehicle controls (e.g. forces, response times, etc.) but on the skills needed to handle the vehicle in all traffic situations.

If one looks however into the directives of vehicle components, several requirements are found with respect to the operation of components, which are directly related to the physical abilities of an "average" person. The assumptions with respect to the functional abilities of the user can preclude (part of) the elderly and disabled population from driving although they might be able to operate the vehicle properly if supported by specially fitted equipment suited to their physical abilities.

The main objective of this paper is to highlight some vehicle design aspects for their consequences with respect to the driving possibilities of elderly and/or disabled (potential) drivers.

Three types of actions can be defined in modifying a vehicle such that it can be adequately controlled by persons with different physical abilities (referred to as "Drivers with Special Needs") compared to the so-called "average" driver. Ordering these actions in priority, one obtains:

- reducing the number of control functions (e.g. automatic clutch or transmission)
- giving assistance by reducing power and/or motion of the control (e.g. power braking, power steering)
- modification, realocation of possibly alternative controls (e.g. hand controls, foot steer)

In this paper, the focus is on the power assistance and/or modification of the longitudinal control of a vehicle (i.e. braking and acceleration) and steering. With respect to power assistance, the main question to be raised is the determination of the proper assistance levels. There is some evidence that more information on the vehicle performance in relation with the driver is needed to avoid unnecessary modification and/or allow for user-critical vehicle comparison. In addition to power assistance to lower the upper limit of the required force by the driver, also the lower limit of assistance in relation to the type of control needs further consideration. Too low control forces compared to for example gravity forces and/or dynamic forces on the operating limb might be difficult to apply, yielding uncontrolled situations as will be demonstrated for braking and steering controls. An important issue that needs to be considered is that if the driver is fully dependend on power assistance to perform part of the driving task, the standard requirements in this case of failure of the system have to be reassessed to ensure an equal safe driving situation.

The main conclusion to be drawn is that vehicle design principles based on the "average" physical abilities of the user need reconsideration in view of a growing elderly and disabled population. This needs to be embedded in clear and complete regulation on legislation on a European level.

1. INTRODUCTION

Mobility plays a key role in everyday life. For most trips like shopping, going to work, visiting relatives or going on holidays, we rely on the car. This holds true even more so for many elderly and disabled people.
However, part of the elderly and disabled population have functional limitations that limit or restrict them in operating a standard car. The main objective of this paper is to highlight some vehicle design aspects for their consequences with respect to the driving possibilities of elderly and/or disabled (potential) drivers. The focus is on the power assistance and/or modification of the longitudinal control of a vehicle (i.e. braking and acceleration) and on steering.

In the Netherlands, in the periode 1986 - 1988 [3], a total number of almost 1.4 million people were identified with at least some kind of mobility restriction. This is approximately 10 % of the total population. Of this 1.4 million people, approximately 6 % have a very serious mobility problem. They cannot go from one place to another without a mobility-aid such as a wheelchair and/or an adapted car. About 20 % of people with restricted mobility fall in the category "seriously restricted". People in this category make often use of mobility-aids such as a walking frame or a rollator. Figure 1 gives an overview in relation to the total population.

The figures in other European countries are quite comparable. It is reported in [11] that the percentage of the population in the European memberstates with visual, hearing, intellectual and mobility impairments vary between 10.0 % and 12.1 %. The percentage of people with a physical impairment related to the upper or lower limbs is in the order of 6 - 7 % of the total population. The number of people within the European Community who have disabilities related to the lower limbs is estimated at 18.7 million. The European population with upper limb impairments is estimated at 6.1 million.

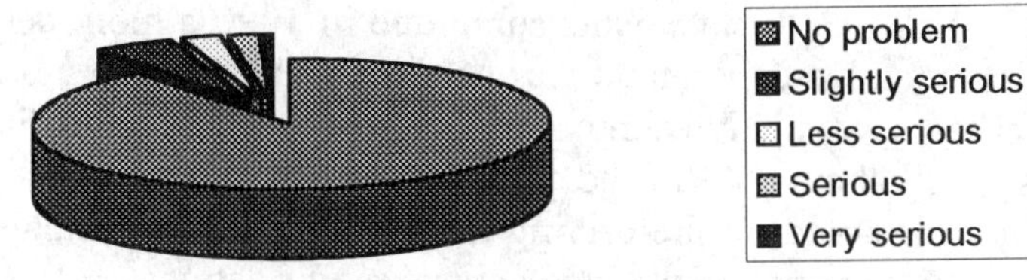

Figure 1.: Mobility problems compared to the total population

What about the car driving population? When applying for the driving licence exam or a renewal of the driving licence, one has to state his medical condition by means of a health declaration. In the Netherlands in 1990, more than 420.000 of these health statements were submitted to the Dutch Driving Licence Authority [15].

About 10% of the health statements were related to the renewal of the driving licence by drivers of 70 years and older. This number will increase steadily over the next years because of the ageing of the population in general and the increased percentage of drivers within the coming generations.

About 30% of all the health statements in 1990 had to be considered by the medical department. Most health problems are related to visual impairments (144.000). About 45% of visual impairments were reported by elderly $\geq$ 70 years. Internal diseases, like diabetes and heart diseases, are frequently reported ($\pm$50.000). About 4000 (potential) drivers reported functional problems of the upper extremities (arm, hand) and over 8000 stated problems with the lower extremities (leg, foot). About 10% and 20% were related to elderly people ($\geq$ 70 years) for problems with respectively the upper and lower extremities.

For 3% of all health statements submitted in 1990 a more detailed assessed by the adaptations department was necessary (14.000). In more than 50% of these cases a practical/technical assessment in relation to the vehicle was necessary. In about 65% of the cases handled by the adaptations department, restraints are noted on the driving licence varying from standard automatic transmission to very complicated control modifications.

The average number of restraints on the driving licence is 2.3 per case [12]. Statistical data over the period 1993 to 1995 shows that the most often used restraints are related to the maximum operating force of the braking system ($\pm$ 25%). Second large are the restraints related to the automatic transmission (18%) and the automatic clutch (17%). Furthermore the adapted steering devices (11%) and adapted accelerator (9%).

It is estimated that about 20.000 to 25.000 cars in the Netherlands are adapted with the more complicated modifications (hand controlled brake, accelerator ring,...), i.e. in the order of 0.5 % of the total number of cars.

Section 2 gives an understanding of drivers with special needs and the way their physical impairments are considered in relation to vehicle handling. Section 3 will focus on the assessment of drivers with special needs. Related regulation in Europe on car adaptation - the European dimension- is discussed in section 4. In section 5 and 6, the mismatches between the potential driving abilities of drivers in a possibly adjusted vehicle and the braking and steering directives are discussed, respectively. Finally, the major conclusions are listed in section 7.

2. DRIVERS WITH SPECIAL NEEDS (ELDERLY AND DISABLED)

There are several reasons for a driver to have "special needs", compared to the average population.
These reasons can be roughly divided into:

- medical impairments and/or diseases (i.e. diabetes, heart diseases, etc.)
- visual impairments (i.e. monocular, poor vision, etc.)

- cognitive impairments (i.e Alzheimer disease, etc.)
- physical impairments (i.e arthritis, spinal cord injury, amputation, multiple sclerosis, etc.)

The medical fitness to drive is determined by medical officers of the driving licence authority based on the health statement submitted by an applicant and/of additional medical consultation(s).
For more details on this process see [7, 10, 13] where relevant literature on this subject is discussed as well as consultation of medical experts in the field are included to arrive at guidelines on the assessment of fitness to drive.

When focusing on the last category, **physical impairments**, in relation to vehicle handling, there are three relevant questions in the health statement for each (potential) driver:

- do you lack the normal use of an arm or hand and/or fingers, or of related joints?
- do you lack the normal use of an leg and/or foot, or of related joints?
- do you suffer other disabilities or illnesses which would hinder or prevent you from driving motor vehicles without special provisions.

These questions should cover all situations in which the physical abilities of the applicant and/or driver are different from the "average" criteria used in vehicle design. The "lack of normal use" can be roughly categorized in:

- missing (part of) limb (i.e. amputation)
- no function of the limb (i.e. spinal cord injury)
- less force application (i.e. arthritis, multiple sclerosis, elderly)
- restricted movement (i.e. arthritis, multiple sclerosis, elderly)
- different reach envelope (i.e. extreme small persons)

In each of these cases, assessment by experts is needed to define what kind of adaptation(s) is needed such that the (potential) driver can cope with a vehicle, currently available on the market. That means that the combination of driver and possible adjusted vehicle is capable to guarantee the same level of safety and driving performance as the "average" driver.

Two typical vehicle adaptations are shown in figures 2 and 3, related to missing upper limbs and missing lower limbs respectively, where the steering control and the brake/acceleration control has to be taken over by the lower limbs and the upper limbs, respectively.

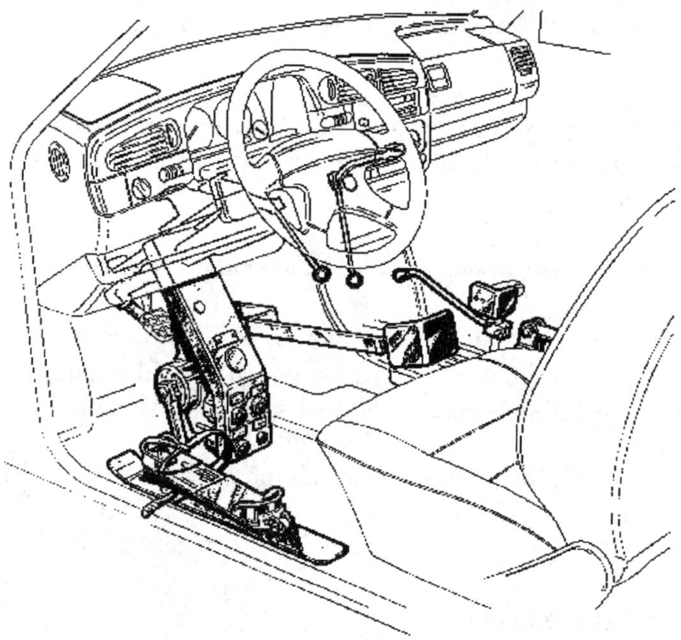

Figure 2.:   **A vehicle adjustment for a driver lacking the function of his/ her upper limbs. (Source: Mobil mit Volkswagen - System Franz)**

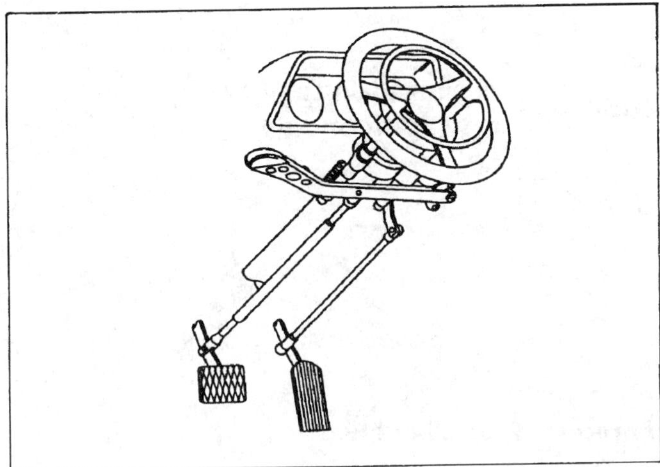

Figure 3.: A vehicle adaptation for a driver lacking the function of his/her lower limbs (accelerator ring on top of steering wheel and manual service brake lever)

3. ASSESSMENT OF DRIVERS WITH SPECIAL NEEDS

Assessment is the first step in the procedure of designing a vehicle adaptation for a driver with special needs, followed by the actual vehicle modification and approval of the car adaptation, as indicated in figure 4. The assessment is done by experts of the adaptations department of the driving licence authority. By combining their expertise as driving licence examiner with their knowledge of the available adaptation possibilities and products, they can define the concept of the necessary adaptation(s). The defined concept will be registered as code(s) on the driving licence. The approval of the modified vehicle is done according to the national regulations in the particular country. Some comments on the (lack of) harmonization within the European community in this respect are made in the next section.

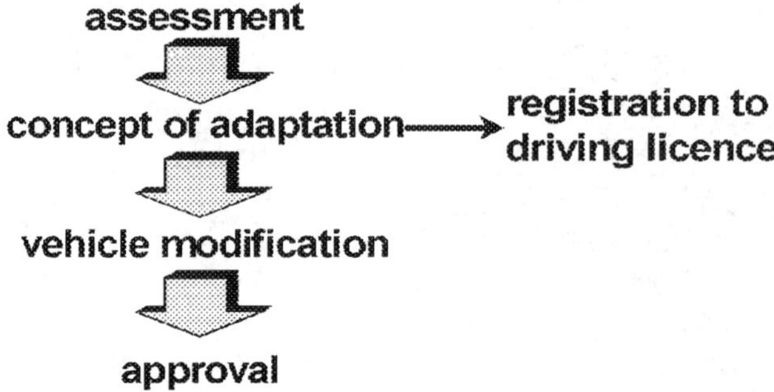

Figure 4.: The general process of car adaptation

Three types of actions can be defined in modifying a vehicle such that it can be adequately controlled by persons with different physical abilities than the "average" (drivers with special needs). Ordered in priority these actions are:

- reducing the number of control functions (i.e. automatic clutch or transmission)
- giving assistance by reducing power and/or motion of the controls (i.e. power braking)
- modification, realocation or alternative controls (i.e. hand controls, foot steer. etc)

The fewer the adaptations the better it is, especially if the financial costs for adaptations are taken into account as well. Therefore the first step is to consider whether, by reducing the number of control functions, the vehicle can be handled by the person involved. Automatic transmission is the best example of reduction of an unnecessary activity. However, the European preconditioning that automatic transmission is only for bunglers gives ground to much less advantageous products as an electronic clutch whereby most of the activity (changing gears) still has to be performed.

As long as the automated highway is not yet reality, each driver has to manage the lateral and longitudinal positioning of the vehicle or in other words: needs to operate the accelerator, brakes and steering mechanism. So these can't be left out like the transmission. The second step is then to see whether the effort needed for these activities can be reduced by power assistance. Power assistance is more and more offered as standard comfort feature, but for some elderly and disabled the degree of assistance needed will be beyond the standard offered level.

In case the (potential) driver doesn't have the functional abilities to operate the (power assisted) controls, the installation of alternative, modified and/or reallocated controls has to be considered. A nearly infinite number of (often custom-made) possibilities are available. Some more general solutions will be given in the following paragraphs.

The driving licence directive [14] gives an outline of the requirements and assessment criteria to determine the medical fitness to drive and the driving skills of the European driver. All drivers must comply to these criteria. This directive distinguishes between driving skills and driving behaviour. With respect to **driving skills**, according to annex II, paragraph 3.2 of this directive, the driver must be able to operate the vehicle including:

- steer
- accelerator
- clutch
- gear change
- hand- and foot brake

under various specific circumstances referring to starting from stand-still, straight-line driving, speed adjustment at cross-section, driving back and forth, turning, parking, etc. The compliance to these requirements is examined by well trained and officially acknowledged experts during the driving licence examination. Looking in more detail to these requirements makes it clear that they are all related to the skills needed to handle the vehicle in different traffic situations. None of these requirements is directly related to any physical measurables in relation to the vehicle controls (e.g. forces).

This is different for directives of vehicle components like brakes, where several requirements are found with respect to the operation of the components which are directly related to the physical abilities of the "average" person. The assumptions with respect to the functional abilities of the user can preclude (part of) the elderly and disabled population from driving a standard production car although they might be able to handle the vehicle properly when fitted with equipment suited to their physical abilities.

4. EUROPEAN REGULATION AND ASSESSMENT FOR CAR ADAPTATIONS

In addition to the discussion on mismatches between automotive design and potential use of vehicle by drivers with special needs, this paragraph includes some notes on the status of regulations related to car adaptations in the different member states. Current discrepancies between the regulation of the different member states may cause travel restrictions for drivers of adapted cars and may yield trade barriers for car-adaptation manufacturers. The travel restrictions may imply for some drivers of adapted cars that they are not entitled to drive with their car in other countries of the European Community. As long as no accidents occur this will seldom become apparent since the actual knowledge how to deal with car-adaptations is often not wide-spread. The trade barriers may imply additional testing of some products as well and some countries might not permit the usage of some products at all.

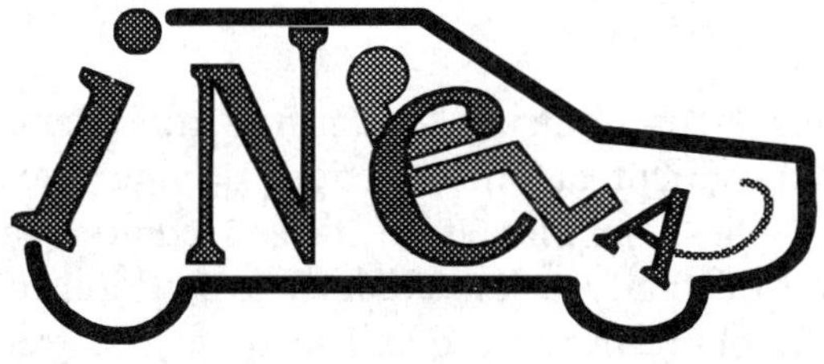

To get insight into this situation at an European level, the **INCA** project has been established by DG VII of the European Commission. INCA is an acronym for an "Inventory of European legislation and regulation for Car-Adaptations", and is carried out under responsibility of TNO. The ultimate goal of the INCA project is to achieve the same level of safety and mobility for disabled people in Europe as for other car users. The first step towards this objective is to identify the actual legislative and regulative situation within the different member states of the European Union. How are the countries currently dealing with car-adaptations and driving by disabled drivers? The second step of the project is the development of a code of practice for car-adaptations and the assessment of the adapted vehicle in relation to the user capabilities. The recommendations in the code will be in line with the rationale of the EC-regulations for standard cars whenever possible.

The present status in Europe can be summarised as follows. After modification of a vehicle, it is in many countries (e.g. Germany, Netherlands, Italy, Belgium) necessary to have the car homologated by the Ministry of Transport before being allowed to drive the car on the public roads. This inspection is often delegated to a special department or organisation but the Ministry of Transport sets the rules and regulations. The inspector will check whether the conversion has been carried out in accordance with the current legislation and/or according to best practice. The modifications should not create any danger for the vehicle occupants or other road users. The inspection criteria are mostly based on or closely related to the European Directives as used in the Type Approval. In a few countries special legislation for car-adaptations for disabled drivers is available. This mostly concerns rules that allow to deviate from specific clauses in the EC-Directives if essential for the control of a system by physically handicapped people. The inspected modifications are written down in the registrations documents of the car. This can vary from 'adapted for usage by disabled driver' to a more detailed description of the type of adaptation.
This situation is quite different in Great Britain, where adaptations and converted vehicles are not inspected and no approval is required from the government. In principle drivers are free to choose the equipment and have it installed by anyone capable to do so. This freedom may sometimes result in installations that lack quality and/or do not provide an optimal driving solution. The driver can get assistance from several assessment centres that give advice on the driving capabilities and suitable adaptations.

In many of the other countries of the EC the choice of the type of adaptation is done by an official expert from either the vehicle inspection or the driving licence authority. The necessary driving adaptations are indicated on the driving licence by means of codes as mentioned earlier. A proposal for harmonisation of these codes has recently been adopted and will be implemented in the coming years.

An overview of the legislative and regulative situation in the different European countries is drafted at the moment and expected to be available around spring next year, as part of the INCA project. An overview of the experts and authorities involved in the field of car-adaptations is also expected around the same time. By the end of 1998, INCA will deliver its first version of the code of practice for the evaluation of car-adaptations.

5. BRAKING

Some of the discrepancies between the braking directives (71/320/EEC) and the use by drivers with special needs are discussed in this section. Examples of such discrepancies are related to the required service force versus the available force, the fail safety in case of for example power assistance failure, the exclusion of electronic brakes, the requirement of not removing the hands from the steering control during braking, etc.

The driving licence directive (91/439/EEC) stipulates that the driver should be able to brake the vehicle properly, and if needed with full brake power (Annex II, article 3.2.6).

The braking directive (71/320/EEC) stipulates performance criteria for brakes of vehicles (Annex II, article 2.1.1). The prescribed braking performance must be obtained by an operating force of maximum 500 N for the service and secondary brake, and a maximum force of 700 N for the residual brake. These forces are (far) beyond the functional abilities of part (in the order of 10-20 %) of the elderly and disabled population. Measurements with arthritis patients showed for example maximum available forces of less than 150 N [2].

The brake performance requirements of the directive are however a pass/fail tests, and very seldom information is given on the actual forces to be applied to the control to pass the requirements. This information would be of great interest for many elderly and disabled (potential) drivers. It would allow a more objective comparison at operational level and could avoid unnecessary adaptation. The importance of this information is underlined by the fact that around 10-25 % of the applicants that are assessed by the experts of the adaptations department get a restriction on their driving licence with respect to operation force of the service brake.

A quick scan through Cardata [1] shows that the brake forces of standard production cars varies quite significantly amongst the market supply. The graph shows some examples of the **operation forces** for the brake of standard production cars. These results are randomly chosen out of the available data and not placed in any order in relation to the mentioned vehicle manufacturers.

When (potential) drivers lack the force to operate the brakes properly as requested in the driving licence directive, the expert of the adaptation department will measure the available operation force at the pedal with a special brake-force measurement device. If this force is lower than 500 N, a code will be registered on the driving licence that clearly shows the maximum operation force of the brake. The code implies that the driving licence is only valid if the person concerned drives a vehicle of which the brake forces comply to the stated level. Note however that the driving licence directive requests for the ability to make an emergency stop. The operating force during an emergency stop (a ~ 8 à 10 m/s^2) will most probably exceed the normally quoted operation force according to the braking directive (a = 5.8 m/ s^2).

Since there is hardly any information available on the vehicle, the vehicle/driver combination is currently checked by making an emergency stop during a driving test.

Service brake force (N)

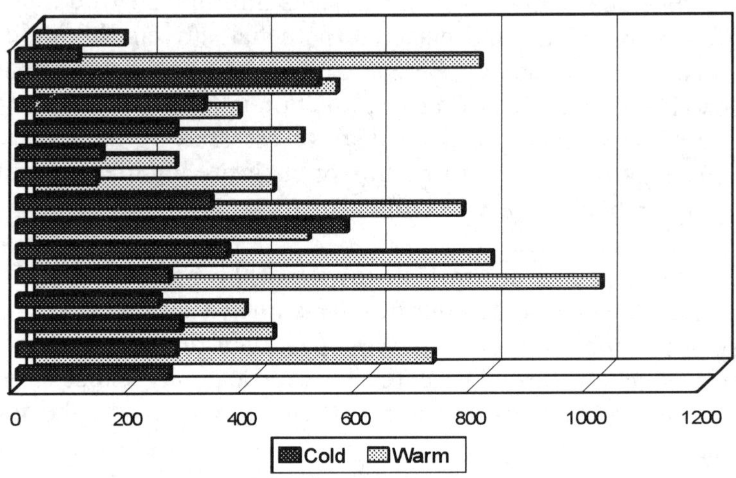

Figure 5.:   Service brake force for some passenger cars, randomly chosen out of the available data [1] of standard production cars from all major vehicle manufactures.

Until now the focus was on the **upper limit** of the brake operating force. There is however also a **lower limit** of the needed control force. Because of the inertia of the (lower) leg, the operation force of an ordinary foot controlled brake pedal should stay above circa 100 N. This figure is based on extensive experience and not on any specific research data. If the available force of the (potential) driver is below this lower limit of 100 N, the use of different types of controls has to be considered. This can in example be a tilted pedal or a pedal by sole. The other possibility is to modify/reallocate the brake function from the foot to the hand by installation of hand controls. For hand operation, the force can be lowered to as low as about 10 N. If going beyond that level, even with modified systems the dynamic forces on the limb will become of such influence that nearly every stop becomes a kind of emergency braking situation.

Another point that needs to be considered when assessing the elderly and disabled drivers is the safety in case of a **system failure**. An "average" person who uses the power assistance for comfort reasons is expected to be able to control the vehicle in case of any power failure. Furthermore the braking directive (71/320/EEC) stipulates the existence of a secondary braking device in case of failure of the service brake and a residual service braking after transmission failure. A disabled and/or elderly driver who completely depends on power assistance for normal operation of the service brake won't be able to control the vehicle in case of power failure nor will he be able to operate the secondary and/or residual braking system. In order to establish equal safety for the "average" as well as the elderly and disabled drivers, back-up systems should be considered for all failure critical elements of a power assisted braking system.

The main category of alternative brake systems is the so-called manually operated service brake. Most of these systems consist of a lever within hand reach that is connected to the original brake pedal by several rods (see figure 3). The actual operation force will in these situations depend on the dimensional design of the rod-system. There are a few electronic brake systems on the market, but they are used only on small scale because of the price level ($\pm$ 5000 ECU) and the fact that electronic brakes are not allowed according to the braking directive. It should be noted that according to the braking directive, it should also be possible to achieve the braking action without removing the hands from the steering control (71/320/EEC, paragraph 2.1.2.1). This is impossible in case of lever type constructions. The operation device of the electronic brake can be placed on the steering wheel to comply with this requirement.

Most cars that are adapted for drivers with special needs **have also to be used by family and/or friends**. Whenever possible the original equipment should stay in place. In case of the installation of a manually operated brake, the brake pedal is usually made fold away or detachable to avoid unintended activation by the legs and/or feet of the driver.

Another point of concern is that in case of (full) power assistance, the brake system should be capable of being **overloaded** in case of emergency reaction of an "average" person.

The last issue to be mentioned with respect to braking systems to the possibility of **combined actuation of brake and accelerator**. Although it is not excluded by control design, we usually expect to operate the pedals such that we don't actuate the acceleration and brake at the same time. In case of a fully manual controlled car with e.g. an accelerator ring on the steering wheel and a separate brake lever this separation has to be included in the design since it can not be implemented in the operation. (The driver will always keep one hand at the steering wheel when using the brake). Especially for drivers with extreme low physical abilities this is of importance since "lifting" of the acceleration requires an active operation which might not be attractive for the driver to put effort in. There are several systems on the market that release the acceleration as soon as the brake is touched. Some also have the feature that the acceleration first has to pass the "neutral" position before it can be actuated again. This to prevent the situation that at release of the brake at stopping position one is not "launched" because the full acceleration due to dynamic forces on or the dead-body weight of the operating limb.

6. STEERING

Steering can be a problem for an elderly or disabled driver for several reasons. Most of the discrepancies for braking as reported in the preceding section apply for steering as well. This may be related to the required steering torque versus the available torque, the use of other than mechanical devices (such as hydraulics or "steering by wire"), the need for back-up systems when power steering is used, etc. A special concern is the position of the steering wheel. We refer to [5] and [6].

The **position of a steering wheel** with respect to the horizontal plane can be critical in the capability of the driver to steer the vehicle. In commercial vehicles, the steering wheel is usually designed more horizontally than in a passenger car. For a tetraplegic being not able to lift his arm sufficiently, such a design will be beneficial. A too upright position can be a serious obstacle for the driver to carry out a steering manoeuvre due to the required arm-motion, even if the required steering torque is very low.

Clearly, a horizontally positioned steering wheel is hard to be mounted in an average passenger car. One might consider a joy-stick steering device, however at the cost of running into some approval problems. Since a joy-stick device normally has no mechanical connection to the wheels, it conflicts legal conditions (70/311/EEC). Steering systems with electric, pneumatic or hydraulic transfer of control and feed-back information between steering device and vehicle motion are not allowed at present, except under special restrictions (e.g. maximum speed).

In [5], data is gathered on required steering torque, with and without power assisted steering for normal production cars, as shown in figure 8.

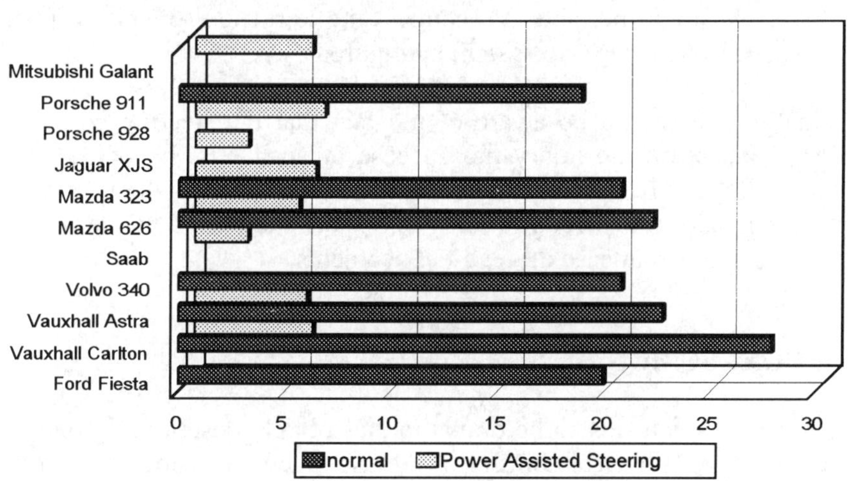

Figure 6.: Required steering torque for some passenger cars

It is reported in [5] that for drivers suffering from multiple sclerosis or spinal difficulties, an available steering torque as low as 5 Nm could be expected, regardless of the available arm-motion. According to figure 8, such a value is quite feasible in case of power assisted steering. Power assisted steering is even available up to a maximum control force as low as 10 N, that means a steering torque of 2 Nm.
Now let's suppose the car is making a sharp bend to the left, resulting in a significant lateral inertiaforce on the steering arm. This could easily be in the order of 10 N, i.e. yielding a steering moment in the order of the required steering torque. Clearly, if the driver is not able to withstand forces in this order of magnitude, uncontrolled behaviour results and, in addition, appropriate feedback of the vehicle heading position through the steering controls is not available. This has to be taken into account, also (and especially) when joy-stick control is considered.

Without such power assisted steering (i.e. if it fails), a maximum steering force of 450 N is allowed [6]. This means that in case of system failure, the driver will not be able to control the direction of his car anymore. Consequently, a back-up system is required.

Finally, one should be aware of the fact that the steering controls have a large impact on the injury-risk in case of accidents. In fact, steer-by-wire would be very beneficial in this respect. More specific, the use of a steering handgrip allows to steer with only one hand but such a handgrip might lead to large injuries in case of head-tail accidents.

7. CONCLUSIONS

The main conclusion to be drawn is that vehicle design principles based on the "average" physical abilities of the user need reconsideration in view of a growing elderly and disabled population. This total population can be estimated in the order of 25 million drivers with special needs within the European Community restricting to disabilities related to lower and upper limbs. A rough indication of the number of adapted cars within the EC amounts half a million.

The first priority in car modification is reduction of control functions, in many situations achieved by using automatic transmission. The negative perception and acceptance in Europe restricts the use of automatic transmission and gives ground for less advantageous products.

Discrepancies between vehicle design principles have been discussed for braking and steering. They relate to both maximum and minimum control force or torque, the need for additional backup systems, the potential benefits of non-mechanical devices (hydraulics, steer or brake by wire, joystick exploitation, etc.), the universal use by cars by both handicapped drivers as well as the non-handicapped and the prevention for overloading, the positioning of the control device, etc.
Not only the forces or torques (required versus available) but also the motion (reach, lifting of arms, etc.) should be accounted for. An issue to be considered but not yet fully understood is the information-feedback through the controls and the (handicapped) driver perception of it, see also [8].

REFERENCES

1   FULLAND, J. (ed.): Cardata 01 GB, Interior measurements of cars: A reference for advisers to elderly and disabled motorists.
        SINTEF, TRL and Dept. of Transport. (1994

2   GERRITSE, A.C.: Stageverslag m.b.t. het ontwerpen van een rolsteun voor reuma patienten (Report on the design of a rolling-support for rheumatism patients)
        Twente University (1986).

3   HEKSTRA, A.C., DIJKHUIS, J.: Kwantificering van de aard en omvang van mobiliteitsproblemen bij gehandicapten. (Quantifying the type and amount of mobility problems for the handicapped). TNO-Report 96.OR.VD.019.1/AH (1996).

4   HEKSTRA, A.C., VEENBAAS, R.: Public Transport for Elderly Users of Personal Mobility Aids.
        In: MOLLENKOPF, H., MARCELLINI, F.: The Outdoor Mobility of Older People - Technology Support and Future Possibilities. European Community Publication, COST A5 "Ageing and Technology". Luxembourg (1997).

5 KEMBER, P.: Strength Abilities of Disabled Drivers and Control Characteristics of Cars. Transport and Road Research and Laboratory. Report 215 (1991).

6 LEMPP, R.: Eignungsbegutachtung von körperbehinderten Fahrerlaubnis-bewerbern und -inhabern. Fahrzeugtechnik und Umrüsttechnik.
TüV Verkehr und Fahrzeug Notiz. Fassung 10/97 (1997).

7 LEWRENZ, H.: Krankheit und Kraftverkehr. Schriftenreihe des Bundesministers für Verkehr - Heft 71. (1992).

8 PAUWELUSSEN, J.P.: Effect of Tyre Handling Characteristics on Driver Judgement of Vehicle Directional Stability.
In: PAUWELUSSEN, J.P.: Understanding Human Monitoring and Assessment. Swets & Zeitlinger (1998)

9 STOPPELENBURG, J., TACKEN, M.: Mobiliteitsproblemen van ouderen in een grootschaliger wordende maatschappij (Mobilityproblems of the Elderly in a Society Growing to a Larger Scale). Trail Researchschool, Delft (1995).

10 TAYLOR, J.S. (ed.): Medical aspects of fitness to drive. A guide for medical practioners.
The medical commission on accident prevention (1995)

11 TETZCHNER, S. VON (ed.): Cost 219, Issues in Telecommunications and Disability. Commission of the European Communities, Luxembourg (1991).

12 VEENBAAS, R.: Analysis of CBR data to define a user population for driving Nr. 1994/04, Den Haag (1994).simulator studies. Part A: Description of the CBR database and general conclusions. TNO-Report 92.OR.VD.048.1/ROV (1992).

13 Medische rijgeschiktheid. Advies van een commissie van de Gezondheidsraad (Advisory report on medical aspects of fitness-to-drive).

14 Driving Licence Directive.
Publication of the European Community 91/439/EEC.

15 CBR Jaarverslag 1990 (CBR Annual review 1990). Stichting CBR. Rijswijk (1991).

Vehicle Performance: J.P. Pauwelussen (ed.) pp. 67-83

The New Brake Assist of Mercedes-Benz Active Driver Support in Emergency Braking Situations

Wolfgang Kiesewetter, Walter Klinkner, Dr. Werner Reichelt and Manfred Steiner

Mercedes-Benz is the first automobile manufacturer in the world to develop an electronically controlled system for reducing stopping distance in emergency situations. It is called Brake Assist (BAS). This system has been standard in S-class and SL-class models since December 1996 and will be available in other Mercedes automobiles by the middle of 1997 - standard, at no extra cost.

The development of Brake Assist is based on the results of Daimler-Benz Research which reveal that in critical situations, car drivers tend to put their foot down fast enough, but not firmly enough, on the brake pedal. In the initial stages of braking, the electronic Brake-Assist system automatically builds up maximum braking pressure within a fraction of a second, thereby considerably reducing the car's stopping distance. After anti-lock brakes (ABS), airbag, acceleration skid control (ASR) and Electronic Stability Program (ESP), Mercedes-Benz is therefore making a further contribution towards improving road safety and reducing accident figures.

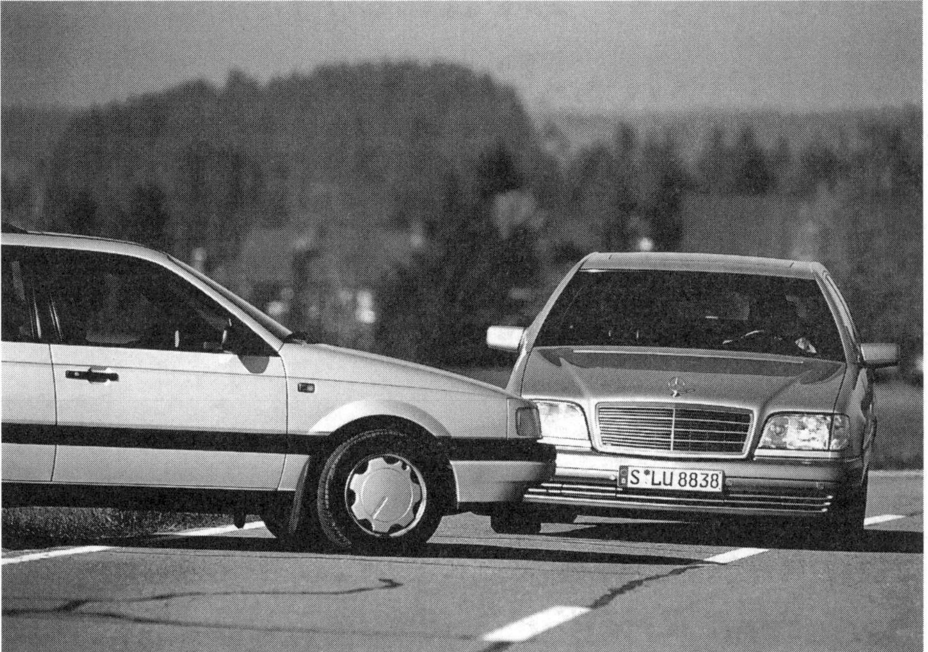

Figure 0: Brake Assist: Braking scene

1. INTRODUCTION

Reducing accident frequency and accident severity is at the center of Daimler-Benz Vehicle Research. In addition to detailed accident analyses, special attention is paid to analyzing the interaction between driver and vehicle. Brake Assist was, for example, developed in the knowledge that rear-end collisions and accidents at junctions account for 50% of all accidents. In most of these accidents, the braking behavior of the drivers involved is at the center of our accident avoidance strategy. Extensive tests were therefore carried out on the driving simulator (**Fig. 1**) in order to obtain precise details of the braking behavior of normal drivers in critical situations. Results impressively confirmed the measurements available at that time from **ZOMOTOR** who, based on a comparatively small random sample, was able to show in particular that normal drivers by no means make maximum use of their vehicle's deceleration potential in critical braking situations.

The intensive analysis of measured data from the driving simulator also revealed that although test drivers do not usually put their foot down firmly enough on the brake pedal and/or do not continue to press the pedal right down after they have started to brake, practically all of them - triggered by a shock reaction in the critical situation - start braking at significantly higher brake pedal speeds than for all other target and deceleration braking actions measured in simulator tests. Brake pedal speeds in emergency braking situations are three times higher on average!

This realization led directly to the idea of Brake Assist - a safe and technically simple means of recognizing the situation in hand. For the first time, driver behavior provided a safe indication of the driver's intended action.

Depending on brake pedal speed, it was now possible to increase braking pressure in conjunction with ABS so that every driver is able to make maximum use of the vehicle's braking potential, even in emergency situations.

Potential studies concerning effectiveness and acceptance were conducted in subsequent driving simulation tests and other field tests using a test vehicle. With a very high level of correlation both on the simulator and in tests performed out on the road, impressive accident prevention potential was revealed (**Fig. 2**): with more than 100 test persons, 84% of "accidents" occurred without but only 16% with Brake Assist.
If the results obtained are compared with forecasts made by **ENKE** on reducing rear-end collisions in road traffic, this produces a reduction potential of almost 50%.

At the same time, evidence was found for an unusually high level of acceptance among normal drivers.

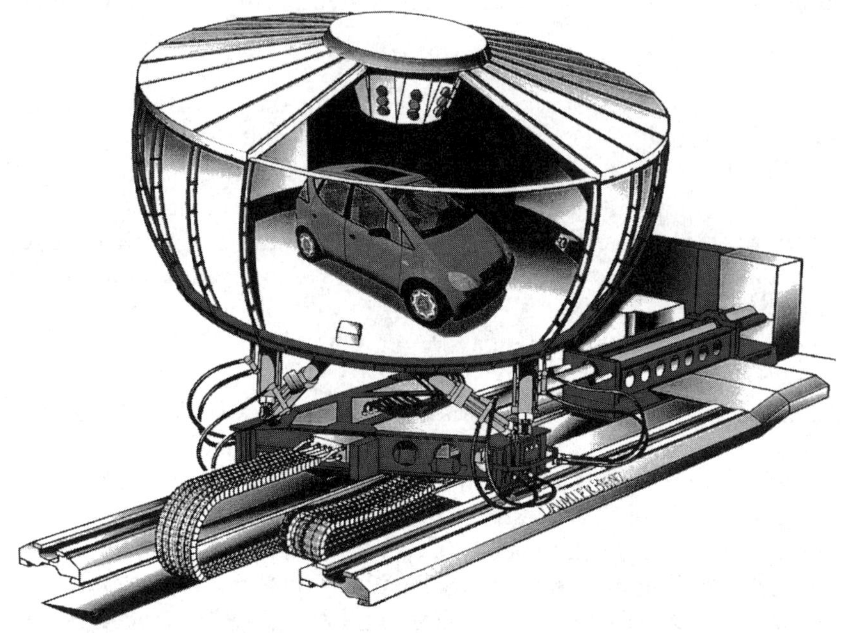

Figure 1: Driving simulator

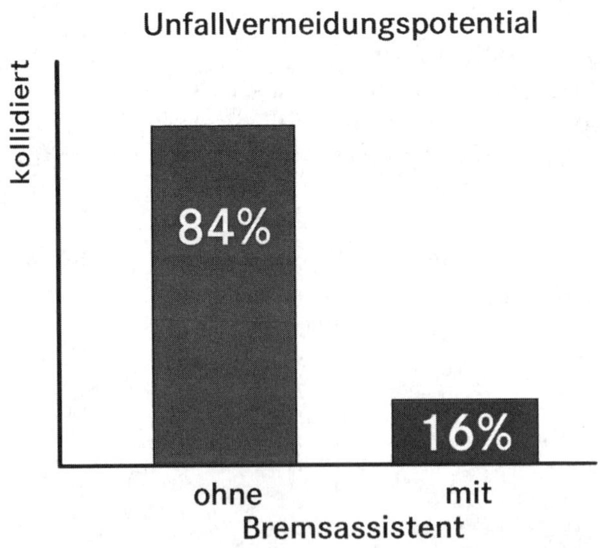

Figure 2: Accident prevention potential of Brake Assist

2. DEVELOPMENT OBJECTIVES FOR BRAKE ASSIST

The most important development objectives of the specifications were:

- Assisting the driver in emergency braking situations, reducing braking time to values which can otherwise only be achieved by drivers with good training.
- Cutting off full brake power as soon as the driver clearly reduces pressure on the brake pedal.
- Retaining the conventional brake booster function. Pedal feel and comfort should meet the usual standards when braking normally.
- Activating the system only in real emergency situations so that the driver does not get too used to it.
- The conventional brakes are not affected if the BAS system fails.
- BAS system failure or non-availability must be displayed to the driver since it would not be obvious during normal driving.
- High availability thanks to optimized and extremely durable electrical and mechanical components.
- Less wiring due to the fact that sensors, actuators and electronics are attached to or installed in the brake booster and that the system is linked up to the CAN data bus.
- Electrical components are to be integrated into and onto the brake booster.
- Standardized control unit and diaphragm travel sensor for all vehicles.
- Low system costs due to the fact that the tried-and-tested, low-cost vacuum brake booster has been retained.
- All Mercedes models fitted with BAS as standard, not an extra; market launch within 6 months in the S-, SL-, E-, C-, CLK- and SLK-class.

3. DESCRIPTION OF BRAKE ASSIST

3.1 Registering the emergency braking situation

The key variable for recognizing the driver's requirement is the speed with which the driver activates the brake pedal (**Fig. 3**). Since the brake pedal and the diaphragm of the brake booster (BKV) are connected mechanically, this variable is deduced from diaphragm travel: a change in diaphragm travel differentiated over a period of time produces diaphragm speed.

While the brake pedal is not activated, the BAS control unit constantly carries out zero point compensation of the travel sensor signal so that the correct actuating travel can be used for calculation during braking.

The Brake Assist logic continually compares actual pedal speed with a threshold value which is constantly adapted to the current situation. If this threshold value is exceeded, the driver requirement "emergency braking" is recognized. In this case, the BAS logic checks various secondary conditions in order to prevent erroneous activation.

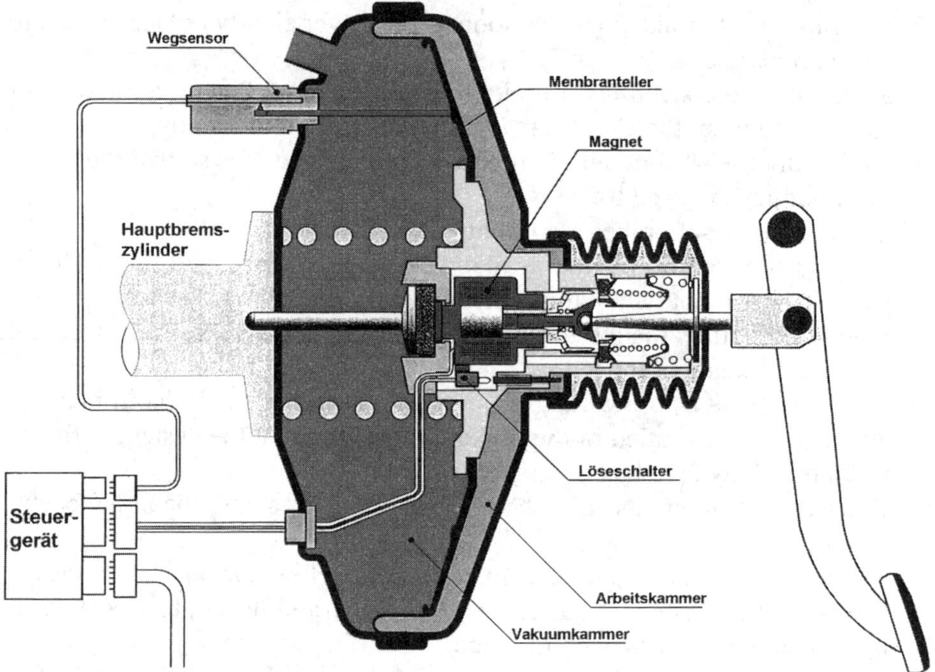

Figure 3: Cross section of brake booster

3.2 Calculating the cut-in threshold

Depending on vehicle speed and actual pedal travel (the driver brakes), the cut-in threshold is dynamically adapted so that the driver's requirements can be recognized safely at any time (**Fig. 4**).

BAS has a choice of parameter sets which are calculated to suit all the differently dimensioned brake systems in the various model series.

In addition, a learning algorithm integrated into the logic takes account of the brake system's current status. Each time the driver brakes, the learning algorithm establishes the relationship between brake pedal travel and vehicle deceleration and compares these values with a specified target characteristic. If certain peripheral conditions are also satisfied, the BAS control unit calculates a correction factor based on the difference between the values actually measured and the target characteristic, via a floating mean value. The peripheral conditions are mainly concerned with the fact that road speed, vehicle deceleration and pedal activation speed lie within certain limits. From this it can be deduced that braking is "normal", without ABS intervention, with medium deceleration and in quasi-steady-state conditions.

Using the correction factor, which influences calculation of the cut-in threshold, differences in brake pedal characteristics are compensated for in such a way that the subjective response sensitivity of the BAS system remains the same throughout the vehicle's complete service life. In addition, the learning algorithm makes it possible to assess the state of the brake system. If the brake system is poorly bled, for example, then greater pedal travel is required to reach a certain vehicle deceleration. This is then expressed in a higher correction factor.

3.3 Engagement of BAS

Once the microcomputer has detected an emergency braking situation, it activates a solenoid valve which immediately lets air into the brake booster,

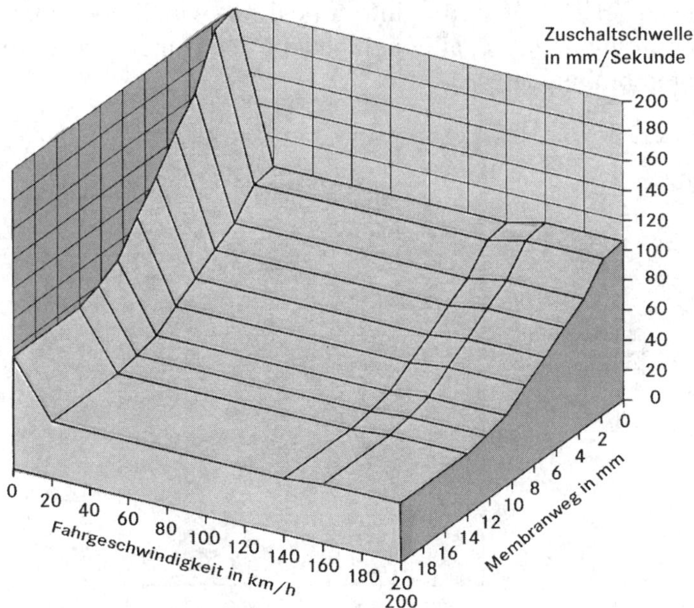

Figure 4: Cut-in threshold as function of diaphragm travel and road speed

thereby building up full braking pressure. Wheel lock is also prevented because ABS continues to meter brake force precisely up to the wheel lock limit, thereby making sure that the car remains steerable.

3.4 Shutting off BAS

The Brake Assist function is shut off by a microswitch (release switch) when the driver reduces pedal force to approx. 20 N, thereby indicating the wish to end emergency braking.
This means that even if pedal force is slightly reduced unintentionally - as was often the case in normal driver tests - BAS support is maintained throughout the entire emergency braking procedure. Pulsation of the brake pedal as a result of ABS control does not cause BAS to shut off either.

3.5 The effect of BAS

Driver support means supplying higher pressure to the brake system than that produced by the pedal power applied by the driver. If necessary, this pressure is built up as quickly as possible and is so great that, with an intact brake system, the wheel lock limit is reached, thereby resulting in ABS control.
The brake pedal, which is rigidly connected to the inlet push rod of the brake booster (BKV), is pulled into a position which corresponds to this very high braking pressure, although pedal force is much lower than purely foot-actuated braking (**Fig. 5**).

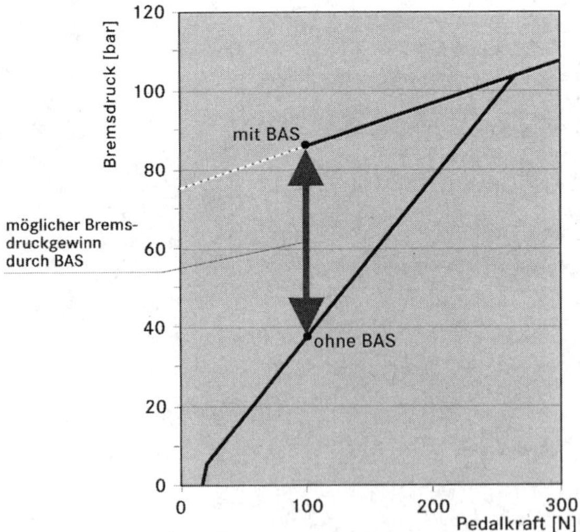

Figure 5: Brake booster characteristic with and without Brake Assist

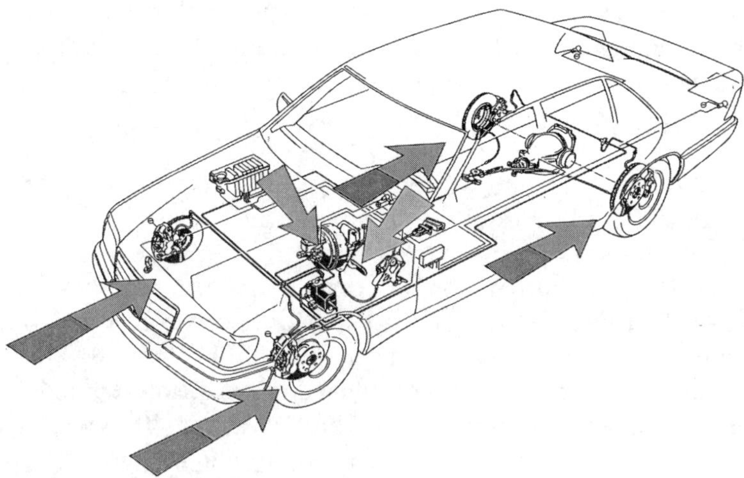

Figure 6: Increased braking power

Despite the low pedal power applied by the driver, high vehicle deceleration is also obvious - the required driver support from BAS. When BAS is activated, braking pressure is clearly increased at all four wheels compared with insufficient braking (**Fig. 6**).

Fig. 7 shows the time diagram of two braking procedures - with and without BAS. Although pedal force is briefly very high due to fast activation of the

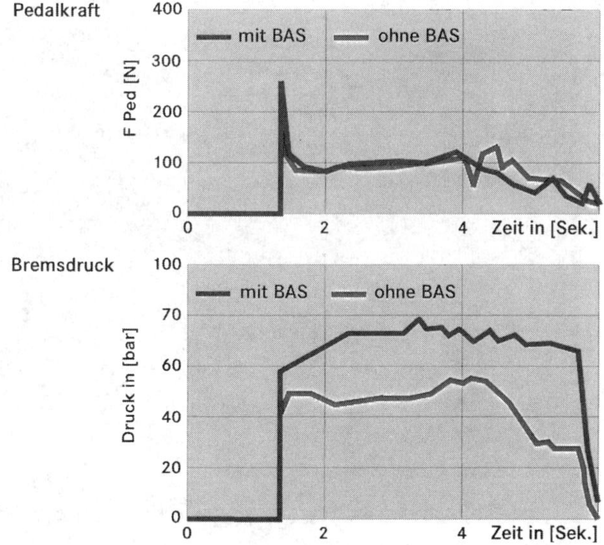

Figure 7: Pedal force and braking pressure

brake pedal, it immediately falls to approx. 100 N which is far too low. At around 65 bar, braking pressure with BAS is much higher than without BAS (around 50 bar). The difference between these two pressure curves is proportional to the gain in stopping distance.

Fig. 8 shows three deceleration variations typical of an emergency braking situation: inadequate driver response, hesitant driver response and the appropriate deceleration variation of a driver with the ideal response or a driver with BAS. The resulting stopping distances are impressive proof of the effect of BAS (**Fig. 9**). On a dry road surface, a driver reacting "inadequately" requires up to 73 meters to brake the car fully from 100 km/h due to the fact that the brake pedal is not pushed down firmly enough. With Brake Assist, the wheels are brought to a halt after just 40 meters, corresponding to a reduction in stopping distance of around 45 percent. Even if the driver only activates full braking power "hesitantly" in the first few seconds, Brake Assist is still able to reduce stopping distance by as much as six meters - more than a car's length.

Incidentally, although this system can drastically reduce stopping distance by optimal braking, it cannot cancel the laws of physics and driving dynamics and their consequences for road traffic.

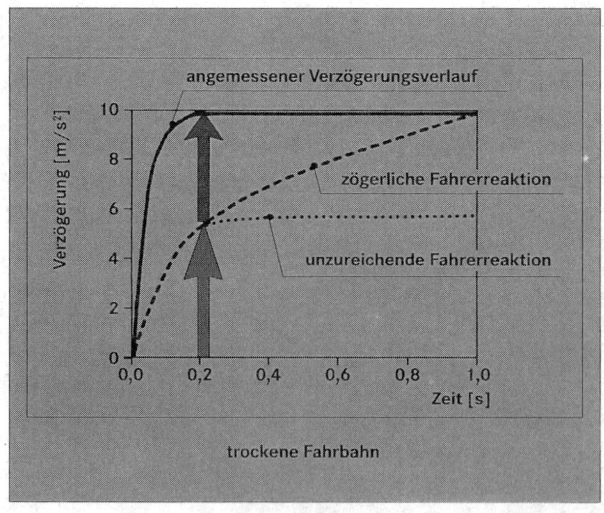

Figure 8: Deceleration variations

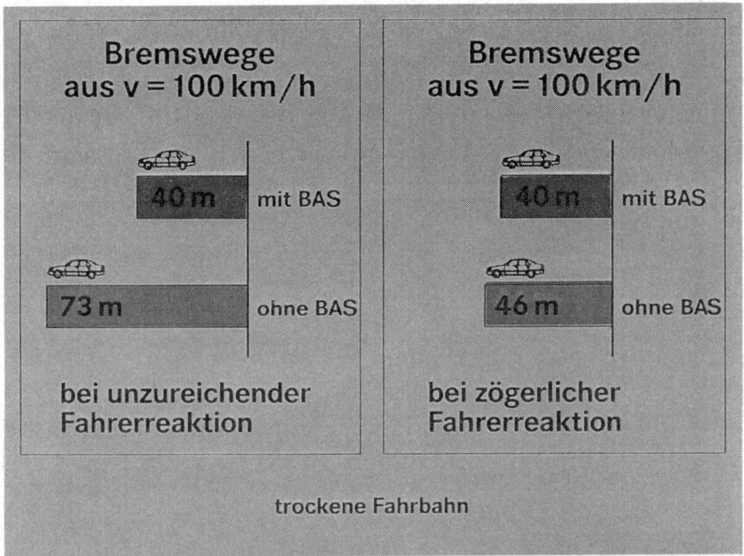

Figure 9: Stopping distance

4. SYSTEM COMPONENTS

The Brake Assist brake booster functions according to the same principle as a conventional brake booster. It is, however, distinguished by four additional components (**Fig. 3**).

- The digitally activated solenoid valve in the brake booster enables its electrical actuation.
- Diaphragm travel is recorded in analog form by the diaphragm travel potentiometer.
- The release switch senses the reduction in pedal pressure.
- The BAS control unit is attached to the brake booster.

The BAS brake booster is therefore a compact unit which can be installed in the same way as a conventional brake booster; only the electrical connection between vehicle and BAS control unit has to be produced additionally.

4.1 Basic function of brake booster

The brake booster, which amplifies the pressure applied to the brake pedal by the driver's foot, consists of two chambers separated by a flexible diaphragm. When the brakes are inactive, there is a vacuum in both chambers. When the brake pedal is actuated, a mechanical control valve in the brake booster is opened so that air flows into the working chamber, thus changing the pressure conditions (**Fig. 30**).

The pressure difference between the two chambers - and therefore the boost power - always corresponds to the instantaneous position of the brake pedal. If the driver only steps gently on the pedal, the pressure difference between the two chambers remains low and the braking effect on the car is correspondingly weak. Maximum boost pressure is obtained when the rear chamber is at full atmospheric pressure. The result is full-power braking. (The brake booster (BKV) is supplied by ITT Industries and Lucas Varity.)

4.2 Electrical activation with solenoid

The control valve which is important for conventional brake boosting can be moved into the full-power braking position by the solenoid. The arma-

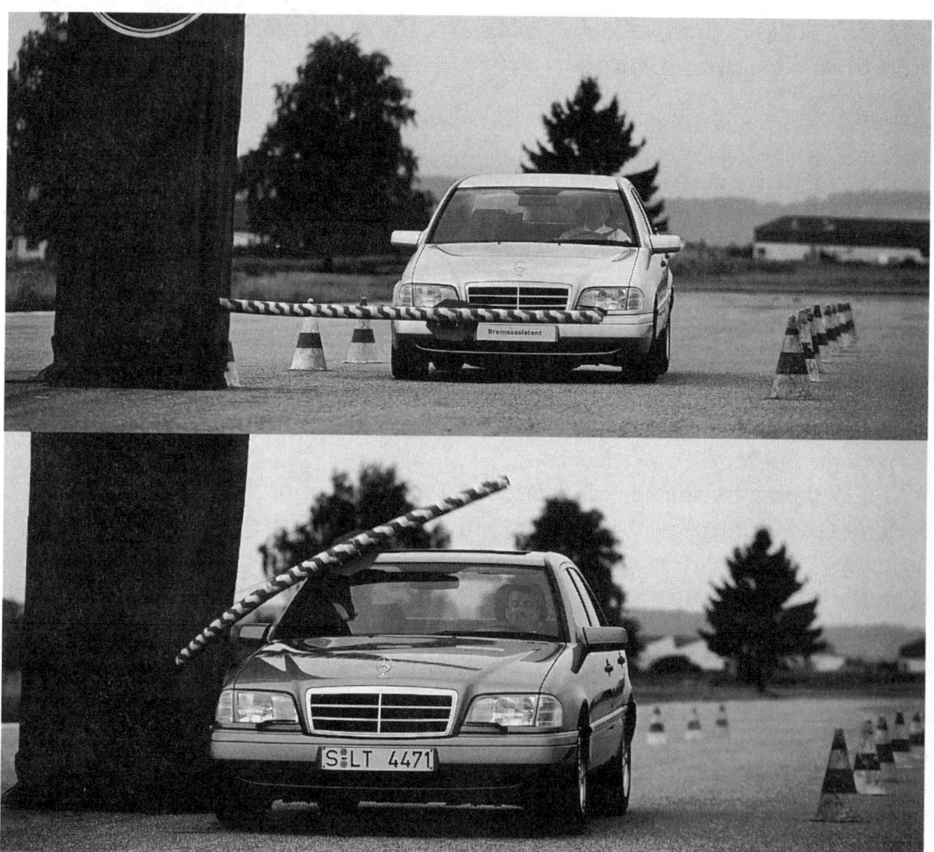

Figure 10:   Field test of emergency braking situation with and without Brake Assist

ture opens the inlet valve and allows air to flow into the working chamber under atmospheric pressure. The brake booster now supplies its maximum possible boost pressure. When the solenoid is deactivated, the brake booster returns to the conventional booster characteristic, i.e. booster pressure is once again proportional to the pedal pressure applied by the driver's foot.

4.3 Diaphragm travel sensor

The diaphragm travel sensor records diaphragm movement proportional to brake pedal travel within the brake booster. This sensor is a resistance potentiometer (manufactured by Helag) which can be used to detect a linear movement of approx. 40 mm. To enable monitoring, it also supplies a certain travel offset in the neutral pedal position and not quite the final potentiometer value when the pedal is pressed right down. In this way, line interruptions and short circuits are easier to identify.

4.4 Release switch

The microswitch integrated inside the brake booster senses when the driver reduces pedal pressure. Following electrically actuated full-power braking, the switch is always activated when the force applied by the driver's foot on the pedal falls below aprox. 20 N. This is the signal for the electronics to deactivate the solenoid valve.

Since it is considered a relevant safety factor for the BAS system to shut off reliably, the release switch is designed as a changeover contact, i.e. electrically redundant. The electronics therefore have access to two separate electric signals which make it possible to check reliably for short circuits and interruptions. The system is designed so that a change in switch signals must take place, even with every normal braking procedure. This means that it is possible to check the plausibility of switch signals at frequent intervals by comparison with diaphragm travel.

4.5 BAS control unit

The electronic control unit (produced by Temic) is also fitted directly to the brake booster. It is responsible for supply, monitoring and signal preparation functions for the diaphragm travel sensor and the release switch. The unit is connected by the CAN data bus to the other electronic systems governing the engine and suspension. This means that wheel speed and the brake light switch are monitored constantly. In addition, each time the engine is started a CAN message is read in for vehicle identification and the suitable BAS parameter set selected accordingly. Only in this way is it possible to use a standardized control unit for all vehicle models and even for two different brake booster suppliers. A single 8-bit microcontroller with integrated CAN processes the input signals and decides every 12 ms whether emergency brake assistance is necessary. For safety reasons, the solenoid valve output stage consists of separate high-side and low-side switches which, in terms of hardware, can only be activated when both release switch signals indicate that pedal pressure has been applied by the driver. Automatic full-power braking without effort on the part of the driver is therefore not possible, even if the electronics are faulty.

The control unit has three watertight plugs, two of which are connected to the travel sensor or the solenoid and release switch directly on the brake booster. The third plug leads to the vehicle wiring harness.

The control unit permanently monitors the sensors and actuators to make sure that permitted voltage levels are not exceeded. In addition, each time the brakes are activated, a safety logic checks the plausibility of sensor signals. If faults to the solenoid valve, release switch, diaphragm travel sensor or the actual electronics are detected, the system is switched to the passive mode. At the same time, a yellow warning light or display in the instrument cluster indicates to the driver that BAS is not available and an entry is made in the diagnosis fault memory.

5. DEVELOPMENT METHODS

Tests were carried out on the driving simulator in Berlin and on test routes to determine the braking behavior of 450 normal drivers. These normal drivers were selected from the public, through newspaper advertisements for example.

Without being warned beforehand, drivers were put into an emergency situation which required powerful braking in order to prevent an accident. In the event of inadequate braking without Brake Assist, the vehicle made contact with the obstacle. The test design is shown in **Fig. 10**.

Extensive road tests were carried out over 5.6 million kilometers for the endurance testing of components and the fine-tuning of logic and parameters. Components had already been subjected by manufacturers to endurance test rig runs under the strictest of conditions, with multiple service life load cycles in some cases. Design, process and system FMEAs were discussed jointly with the companies involved. The process FMEAs were coordinated at suppliers' plants; the system FMEA was carried out by Mercedes-Benz.

Due to its continuity and clearly defined areas of responsibility, the development of BAS is considered a prime example of the development process within Daimler-Benz. First of all, ideas were compiled in research, then, in advance development, they were converted into a purposeful concept suitable for series introduction and finally made ready for series production.

6. COOPERATION WITH THE SUPPLIERS LUCAS-VARITY, ITT INDUSTRIES AND TEMIC

The realization of complex technology with completely new functions, reduced development time and cost optimization calls for a new form of cooperation between supplier and automobile manufacturer. As a rule, Mercedes-Benz applies a form of cooperation known as "Tandem", which has the objective of "Shaping the Future Together".

Within the BAS project, reliability and, above all, fairness in inter-company dealings were applied on a daily basis and at every meeting. Project teams and project managers were appointed as early as the advance development phase. The work of the inter-company project teams was effective. In addition, at the beginning of the series development phase, the "Round Table" committee was set up in which the four project managers and the team members concerned from Mercedes-Benz, ITT Industries, Lucas Varity and Temic regularly reached joint decisions.

Thanks to these very important features, the start-up program, which is unique in terms of time and scope, was realized on schedule at three different Mercedes-Benz production plants.

This is particularly remarkable in view of the fact that outside the BAS project, ITT Industries and Lucas Varity are competitors. Practical results include the awarding of a license for a key feature of the brake booster, and an identical control unit and potentiometer in both suppliers' brake boosters. ITT Industries and Lucas Varity are both system suppliers of the BAS system.

7. OUTLOOK

7.1 Series introduction of Brake Assist by Mercedes-Benz

BAS is to be fitted as standard in the following Mercedes-Benz models at no extra charge: its market launch took place
in the S and SL-class in December 1996,
in the E-class in March 1997,
in the C-class, CLK and SLK in June 1997.

A- and M-class models will follow in 1998 (BAS only in combination with ESP).

7.2 Electronic Stability Program with charging by the Brake Assist brake booster

The Brake Assist brake booster has been further developed so that in addition to full braking pressure, lower braking pressure suitable for charging the ESP hydraulic unit can be produced quickly and at an acceptable noise level. This removes the need for expensive and heavy hydraulic components. Since fewer components are used, ESP system reliability and availability is increased.

The new ESP is to be launched on the market in the E-class in March or April 1997 and in the C-class and CLK in June 1997.

7.3 Proximity-controlled cruise control with proportional pressure build-up by the Brake Assist brake booster

During proximity control, deceleration is built up by engine and possibly brake intervention. Brake intervention must meet the highest demands where comfort is concerned. Brake Assist is therefore fitted with a quasi-proportional solenoid. This is also used in ESP and BAS.

The market launch will take place in the new S-class in 1998.

8. CLOSING REMARKS

Mercedes-Benz is the first automobile manufacturer in the world to develop Brake Assist and launch it on the market. Although Daimler-Benz holds the basic patents to BAS, Mercedes-Benz advocates that the availability of BAS be increased after a lead time of one year. Other manufacturers should then also be able to use BAS.

Mercedes-Benz and all other automobile manufacturers are responsible for making use of all that is technically feasible, with the aim of helping to reduce accident figures. Brake Assist can make a major contribution towards achieving this aim.

REFERENCES

Dr. Zomotor, A.: Fahrwerktechnik: Fahrverhalten, Würzburg: Vogel Buchverlag, 1987

Enke, K.: Möglichkeiten zur Verbesserung der aktiven Sicherheit innerhalb des Regelkreises Fahrer-Fahrzeug-Umgebung, Paris, 7th International Technical Conference on Experimental Safety Vehicles, 1979

Dr. Burckhardt, M.: Fahrwerktechnik: Bremsdynamik und Pkw-Bremsanlagen, Würzburg: Vogel Buchverlag, 1991

Mercedes-Benz Press Department, press information on driving dynamics workshop 1994, Stuttgart, Mercedes-Benz AG, 1994

Dr. Reichelt, W.: Funktion, Wirksamkeit und Akzeptanz von Fahrerassistenzsystemen für kritische Fahrsituationen, Stuttgart, Mercedes-Benz AG, Technical Report (1989) (unpublished)

Dr. Reichelt, W.: Verträglichkeitsuntersuchung von Fahrerassistenzsystemen in Problemsituationen, Stuttgart, Mercedes-Benz AG, Technical Report (1990) (unpublished)

Dr. Reichelt, W., Steiner, M., Kiesewetter, W.: Feldversuch zur Wirksamkeit und Akzeptanz des Bremsassistenten, Stuttgart, Mercedes-Benz AG, Technical Report (1992) (unpublished)

Rump, S.: Feldversuch zur Wirksamkeit des pneumatischen Bremsassistenten, Stuttgart, Mercedes-Benz AG, Technical Report, 1993 (unpublished)

Coermann, G.: Aufbau und Erprobung des Systems Bremsassistent in einem PKW, Stuttgart, University Institute for Internal Combustion Engines and Automotive Engineering, dissertation, carried out at Mercedes-Benz, 1992

Fuchs, A,; Konzeptabsicherung für ein Notfallbremssystem (Bremsassistent), Esslingen, Technical College of Higher Education, report on semester of practical training, carried out at Mercedes-Benz, 1994

Hannus, T.: Untersuchung zum Bremsverhalten von Normalfahrern mit einem Notfallbremssystem, Kaiserslautern, University Institute for Engines and Machines, dissertation, carried out at Mercedes-Benz, 1994

Fuchs, A.: Untersuchung zum Normalfahrerverhalten bei abgebrochenen Notbremssituationen im Fahrsimulator, Esslingen, Technical College of Higher Education, dissertation, carried out at Mercedes-Benz, 1994

Session:

Methodologies

Vehicle Performance: J.P. Pauwelussen (ed.) pp. 87-96

Vehicle Dynamics and the Judgement of Quality

R. S. Sharp

The paper is concerned with the objective specification of required vehicle dynamics qualities, in such a way that meeting the objectives specified will guarantee good subjective reaction to those aspects of the vehicle behaviour which are within the envelope of concern. Two basic types of vehicle dynamics problems are distinguished, one being essentially a machine problem while the other is distinctly a man-machine problem. The current status of quality judging is outlined and its shortcomings are exposed. The basic nature of the driving activity is discussed and a framework for the specification of what is required of the vehicle to be most amenable to the needs of the man is put forward. This leads to some ideas about research directions and improved industrial practices for the future.

1. INTRODUCTION

An improved basis for objectively specifying the behavioural qualities required of a road vehicle, in order for subjects to rate the vehicles highly in a subjective sense, is needed. The effectiveness of virtual vehicle dynamics prototyping is prejudiced by the difficulty, in some fairly high proportion of instances, of deciding what constitutes the best behaviour and conversely. As is well known, the full benefits of concurrent engineering practices include minimum cost product development, fastest to market performance and most nearly right first time products. The prize for fully extending predictive capabilities, extending into proper quality judgements, is great.

A current approach to making progress on the issues is to conduct vehicle tests with instrumentation and to collect subjective assessment results from those same tests [1]. The objective results are then characterised by abstracting certain and often arbitrary performance indicators and using statistical analyses to find which of the selected objective measures best correlate with the subjective assessments. The presumption then is that the correlations obtained are characteristic of the subject area and can be relied upon to distinguish between good and bad performance. This is an approach which is periodically revisited [2, 3, 4]. It is almost bound to yield some impressive correlations but the historical record indicates that the correlations do not constitute understanding, that the arbitrary data reduction process used is questionable, that the picture generated is extremely complicated, that application of the correlation results outside of the immediate circumstances in which they were derived is an enormous act of faith and that re-running the experiments to test their repeatability is too expensive and their reliability remains questionable. Objective indicators of quality have found their way into common application only when there is a sound fundamental basis of understanding for them.

A more fundamental approach is sought, based on consideration of man-machine interaction processes, with driving a vehicle foremost in mind. We distinguish two types of vehicle dynamics problem: One is of input / system / output nature with no man-machine interaction. The ride comfort problem is mainly of this type. It can be characterised by involving a disturbance input which is applied to the vehicle, the ideal response of which would be zero or, if not zero, would have some qualities in keeping with its style. In the simplest terms, we would like the vehicle to be as near a perfect vibration isolator as possible. This is also true in relation to disturbances in lateral and longitudinal directions, which concern the handling problem and which arise from cross-winds and road irregularities. The other concerns substantial man-machine interactions, so that the full problem must be seen as involving a closed loop system, with the man acting as sensing, controlling and actuating systems and the machine responding to the control inputs. The combination of man and machine determines whether or not the sensing, controlling and actuation experiences are satisfying to the man or not. Understanding the man-machine interactions is crucial to making progress with the quality issues in this second type of problem. That is now the focus.

2. CURRENT PRACTICE

A good deal of conventional wisdom in vehicle dynamics is contained in procedures for testing prototypes to determine their suitability for the marketplace. A wide spectrum of different tests is carried out, in a particular sequence, which may be determined by chance or by design. The spectrum of tests is devised to cover all significant aspects of the behaviour, with each individual test having one or more points of focus concerning quality. The main test outcomes are subjective quality ratings and descriptions in an agreed language of the behavioural observations made. Some tests may involve instrumentation and data recording, in which case, the recorded results will, at some stage, be converted into quality judgements by some process which is not globally standardised. Unacceptable weaknesses observed lead to design modifications, which, in principle, will cause changes to all previous test results and will require re-working of much prior testing. Such iterative engineering in practice is slow and expensive and it is bound to lead to quality compromises.

To illustrate the testing procedures, a few examples can be used:

(a) Long wave pitching surfaces are sometimes included in proving grounds. A car traversing such a surface at an appropriate speed will have its body bounce and / or pitch modes excited in resonance and the response level will give an accurate indication of the damping factors of these modes. Large excursions of the suspension will bring the limit stops into play and the progressive nature of their action will be revealed.

(b) Ride comfort on very smooth surfaces is tested for, despite the fact that the road obviously provides very little excitation. The main point of the test is for suspension friction. The very low level of road excitation promotes the friction locking of the suspension. The characteristic motion of the vehicle body with the suspension locked is to resonate with frequency about 4Hz on the elasticity of the tyres, very low energy dissipation being characteristic of tyre deformations. This motion can be felt quite easily, due to its narrow band nature and the absence of other activities.

(c) Steady turning tests on a flat steering pad are used to determine steering angle and steering torque inputs, body roll and the front to rear tyre force balance as functions of lateral acceleration. The steering angle relates to the convenience of the driver in providing the input, while the torque relates to the muscular effort needed. The tyre force balance relates to the static stability and yaw damping (via the understeer level).

(d) An on-centre steering response test operates in a regime in which steering system friction and / or backlash have relatively large influences on the vehicle behaviour. Such features may make the difference between steering wheel torque information responding to tyre / road contact friction level changes getting through to the driver or not. Thus the steer angle / yaw rate, steer torque / yaw rate and steer angle / steer torque relationships may be observed to assess the quality.

(e) The lateral acceleration, yaw rate and roll rate frequency responses to steer angle and steer torque inputs may be determined in a standard linear system frequency response test. The excitation levels used will be large enough for the small amplitude dominant non-linear features like friction and backlash to be negligible but not large enough for the main saturation non-linearity, tyre force saturation, to be influential. In this mid-amplitude range, the frequency response test is the most efficient process for system characterisation. However, it is a matter of conjecture what responses are ideal.

(f) A slalom test may be conducted to examine the roll resonant condition and challenge the overturning immunity of a vehicle. Appropriate speed and wavelength combinations will have to be established in each case to obtain roll resonance and tyre force limiting together. Results relate simply to the adequacy of the damping of the body rolling mode and to the stability of the vehicle in roll. It is conventional wisdom that it is better to slide in the limit than to overturn.

(g) The damping factor of the free control mode may be found by setting a vehicle speed, perturbing the straight ahead motion, and observing the decay of free oscillations. A typical performance criterion would be that there is more than some minimum acceptable damping factor, judged largely from experience.

(h) A test for torque steer may be conducted. From a steady motion condition, the engine throttle would be fully and suddenly opened, with the steering wheel position held fixed. The lateral motion deviation of the vehicle would be an inverse measure of the quality. Braking and / or throttling back in the middle of a steady turn (with fixed steering), with observation of the yaw rate deviation resulting, is a variation on the torque steer test.

The contention is that the whole process discussed and illustrated by these examples has a fundamental pattern to it, which can be revealed by reference to the basics of man-machine interaction dynamics, with special reference to driving.

3. MAN AND MACHINE

Optimal linear quadratic preview control is thought to provide a good model for skilled driving. The application of this theory to suspension control is discussed in [5]. According to this theory, the driver notionally extends forwards from his vehicle a long optical lever and monitors the intended path, in relation to the optical lever, at discrete intervals (operating in discrete time, in which the thinking is simpler) out along the lever, to a distance at which the information is of no current value to him. Note that optimal preview control involves diminishing returns from additional preview and there comes a point when the preview is sufficient for the present purpose. In the case of a single control input, each sample value of the previewed path error, along the intended path, is multiplied by a gain, the gain value corresponding to the sample value position along the previewed path. That is, if 100 sample values, with a 1m sampling interval, making for 100m preview in total, are being used, a particular gain value characteristic of the vehicle, its speed and the cost criterion used in the optimisation will belong to the first sample value, another will belong to the second and so on, up to the 100th value. The sum of the sample value / gain products constitutes that part of the control demand signal which derives from the preview. The total control demand is obtained by addition to this signal of the feedback component, which is the same as that from a non-preview full state feedback linear quadratic optimal controller. It is surmised that what the driver does in the vehicle dynamics learning phase is to work out these optimal gains as functions of vehicle speed, so that he can subsequently perform as the optimal controller. Optimal linear preview control is illustrated in Fig.1. Non-linear behaviour of the vehicle will clearly complicate the necessary activity. Nevertheless, this model of driving and of driving skills acquisition is considered a useful basis for further thinking and deduction.

In the learned state then, the driver previews the path, applies the skill described to convert the path information into a steering angle demand and, if everything works out perfectly and the path intended is followed precisely, no further activity is needed. In the event of an imperfect path following, feedback control has to be utilised to reduce errors. This is harder work than preview control and the driver's preference will be for maximum success from the preview control and minimum need for feedback control. Thus, anything that can be done in the engineering of the vehicle to enhance the effectiveness of the preview control will raise the quality and conversely.

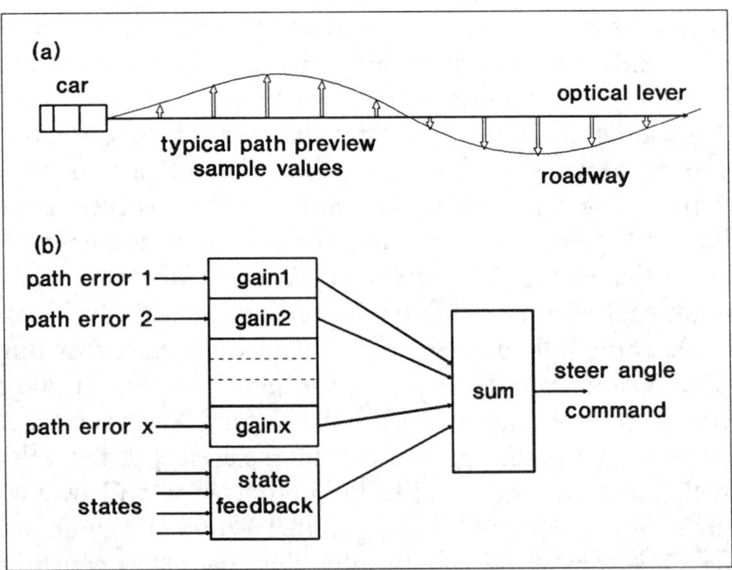

Figure 1: Illustration of the working of optimal linear quadratic preview control. (a) shows the collection of path information; (b) shows the control strategy.

4. VEHICLE REQUIREMENTS

On the basis of the above arguments, a tentative list of vehicle qualities can be written down:

(a) Stability: Characteristic instabilities of vehicles include static yaw instability associated with oversteering and high speed, overturning instability, steering shimmy, car / trailer combination snaking, wobble and weave of motorcycles etc. Static instability of the machine obliges the man to provide continuous stabilising control. The workload implied is bound to be considered disadvantageous. With dynamic instabilities which are not controllable by the man, the man-machine system is likely to meet with disaster. With those which are, the requirement on the driver to provide stabilisation of the system will be a problem as before.

(b) Damping of oscillatory modes of motion: Underdamped modes of motion will generally be excited by driver control and possibly disturbance inputs and, if they are not damped actively, will cause the vehicle motion to be oscillatory. The driver will prefer a well damped motion and may well be able to obtain it by providing damping actively. The controllability of the underdamped mode with respect to steering wheel or longitudinal control input will determine the feasibility of providing damping actively. However, the workload implied is again a disadvantage.

(c) Attitude maintenance: The driver makes observations of the environment continuously from the moving platform of the vehicle. Particularly, the orientation of the vehicle body affects the complexity of the view which he obtains. Excessive pitching, for example, will make the obtaining of path preview information relatively complicated. The ideal from the point of view of accurate sensing with minimum effort is to ensure the minimum rotational response of the vehicle body to disturbance inputs. Zero roll cornering is well liked by those who have been able to try it.

(d) Response delay: Long delays between command input and vehicle response is known to be problematic. In the automotive context, substantial delays have been experienced with turbocharged engines responding to throttle control by first building up the boost pressure and only later raising the engine torque. It is likely that the loss of quality associated with lags is related to the lag time in a highly non-linear fashion, such that very short lags have only a small cost while long lags are quite intolerable. It would be advantageous to be able to quantify the lag time / loss of quality relationship.

(e) Cross-coupling: A vehicle has two basic control inputs; the throttle / brake, primarily for longitudinal control and the steering for lateral control. If the lateral response to longitudinal control and the longitudinal response to lateral control are nil, the control problem is simplified in comparison with the general cross-coupled one. Torque steer is a common undesirable phenomenon in this category. On the other hand, one of the limitations of a front only steered vehicle is that control of the rear tyre forces cannot be exercised directly but only through the reaction of the rear axle to steering of the front wheels, via the body motions. Consequently, it can be useful and attractive, especially to the more highly skilled and interested driver, to have the ability to influence the rear tyre forces via throttle control. This can be done with higher powered rear wheel drive cars, once they are established in a corner. Two basic types of driver can be imagined, the one preferring the controls to be as simple as possible, the other being prepared to accommodate greater complication if this is accompanied by extended performance possibilities.

(f) Output correlations: The steering control problem, decoupled from the longitudinal control problem, involves only one control input, that from the steering wheel. Even with the simplest vehicle, there are two outputs of interest, the lateral acceleration and the yaw rate. In a more general case, the roll angle may also be considered a significant response. Clearly, the possibility of conflicts arises in cases where there are several system outputs, with only one input by which to control them. The control input which forces one response to be that desired, may cause another output to be in error. If the vehicle dynamics can be so arranged that the outputs are correlated, the control input which is ideal from the point of view of one output can be made ideal from the point of view of the others too. It is possible that advantages gained from rear steering control have arisen from this mechanism, popular control laws being those which minimise phase differences between lateral acceleration response and yaw rate response.

(g) Behavioural consistency: Since skilled driving is learned and effective learning is encouraged by task consistency, it is desirable that vehicles are as consistent in their responses as possible. Thus it can be argued that large changes in response with input frequency, in a frequency response test, with vehicle speed, loading, road surface texture, ambient temperature, lateral acceleration level etc. are undesirable.   They will prejudice easy and accurate learning. Nevertheless, it is inevitable that vehicles have performance limited by saturation of the tyres. This makes it not possible to have totally consistent vehicle properties over all running conditions. In such a situation, the best that can be done is that the vehicle behaviour changes progressively as the limit is approached and that there is some information provided to the driver by the vehicle behaviour which is a reliable indicator of the closeness of the saturation limit to the present running condition.

(h) Control quality: For learning to be most effective, control input and vehicle response should have the maximal, sustained relationship to each other. If, for instance, a control input chain contains backlash or friction, some of the movement, in the first case, and some of the control force in the second, will be related to the backlash or friction and not to the system responses. Control systems containing hysteretic elements will give multiple valued relationships between input and response, with dependence on the history of the motions occurring. These features will prejudice easy and effortless learning. Thus it can be concluded that such properties in the control chain are undesirable and that methods for measurement of the strength of relationship between input and output, for example cross-correlation function calculations, will be of interest.

(i) Performance envelope: Other things being equal, bearing in mind that vehicles and drivers share the road space with other such combinations and to some extent compete against them, as wide a performance envelope as possible is desirable. A wide envelope will probably encourage not operating too close to the physical limits of performance and is likely to promote a sense of satisfaction with the vehicle. It may be fundamental to the engineering of the vehicle that extending the performance envelope is in conflict with the progressiveness of the saturation behaviour, in which case, a compromise would have to be struck between two conflicting ideals.

5. FURTHER WORK

The ideas exposed above are hypotheses at the present time. They lead naturally to the idea that research of a hypothesis testing nature is needed, in order to establish, modify or disprove the hypotheses. Since the crux of the arguments is to do with man-machine interaction dynamics, experiments in this area are clearly necessary.   Work is proceeding to design suitable experiments, with the hope that the ideas will survive critical scrutiny.

REFERENCES

1. Chen, D. C. and Crolla, D. A., Subjective and objective measures of vehicle handling: Drivers, Experiments, Simulation, Proc. 15th IAVSD Symposium on The Dynamics of Vehicles on roads and on tracks (L. Palkovics ed.), Budapest, Aug. 1997, in printing.
2. Lincke, W., Richter, B. and Schmidt, R., Simulation and measurements of driver vehicle handling performance, SAE 730489, 1973.
3. Bergman, W., Measurement and subjective evaluation of vehicle handling, SAE 730492, 1973.
4. Jaksch, F. O., Driver-vehicle interaction with respect to steering controllability, Proc. 5th IAVSD Symposium on The Dynamics of Vehicles on roads and on tracks (A. Slibar and H. Springer eds), Swets and Zeitlinger, 1978, 301-319.
5. Sharp, R. S., Preview control of active suspensions, Smart Vehicles (J. P. Pauwelussen and H. B. Pacejka eds), Swets and Zeitlinger, Lisse, 1995, 166-182.

Vehicle Performance: J.P. Pauwelussen (ed.) pp. 97-120

Subjective and Objective Assessment of Manual, Supported, and Automated Vehicle Control

**A.P. de Vos, J. Godthelp,
W.-D. Käppler**

In this paper subjective and objective assessments of vehicle control are illustrated by means of experiments concerning manipulation of vehicle dynamics, driver support, and automated driving. Subjective ratings are discussed in relation to objective performance measures.

The relationship between driver opinion of vehicle handling characteristics and objective measures has been studied. Handling conditions were manipulated by means of varying tyre pressure and lane width. Subjective assessments were determined by means of a two level rating scale. Drivers were found to compensate for varying handling conditions, maintaining a constant performance level by adapting their steering effort. The objective performance measure Time-to-line-crossing (TLC) proved to be a valid predictor for subjective ratings. Changes in vehicle dynamics did not influence visual sampling strategy as derived from a visual occlusion technique.

It was found that active steering support reduced visual workload and improved steering performance, with small effects on steering strategy and steering effort.

Finally, the subjective assessment of fully automated driving in traffic lanes of varying configuration showed that a physical separation between lanes did not affect comfort when driving under automated control, but it was a discomfort factor in manual driving. Driving in the same lane conditions manually, subjects chose speed reduction over increasing steering effort to maintain the proper level of performance.

1. INTRODUCTION

There is a constant development in making cars safer and more comfortable through improved handling characteristics and through new systems that support drivers or even take over (parts of) the driving task. Such developments include the evaluation of handling properties, driver workload and comfort in relation to system characteristics.

In this paper it is discussed how subjective ratings of handling characteristics are correlated to Occlusion time and Time-to-Line-Crossing (TLC) [4]. Occlusion time, i.e. the time that a driver does not need to look at the road for proper lane keeping can be used as an indicator for visual workload. TLC is an objective performance measure which incorporates characteristics of the vehicle, the road and the driver. The impact of a driver support system on these objective measures is discussed [12] and finally the subjective assessment of different characteristics for an automated traffic system is described [9].

2. SUBJECTIVE AND OBJECTIVE ASSESSMENT OF VEHICLE DYNAMICS

Because of driver adaptation processes, performance data such as lateral deviation with respect to the intended course show only minor influences of task difficulty as affected by e.g. road geometry or vehicle dynamics. Performance data are therefore less suitable for predicting driver assessments. Studies by Godthelp and Käppler [4] have shown that the Time-to-Line-Crossing (TLC) as developed by Godthelp, Milgram and Blaauw [2] is a powerful system performance measure that quantifies the time available to the driver for neglecting path errors. TLC is based on a predictor model and represents the time necessary for a vehicle to reach either edge of the driving lane, assuming a fixed steering strategy during the time span of the prediction. Fig. 1 gives a schematic presentation of the path predictions made in such a model. TLC is sensitive to handling differences and therefore it was analyzed whether TLC might serve as a valid predictor of assessment with cars.

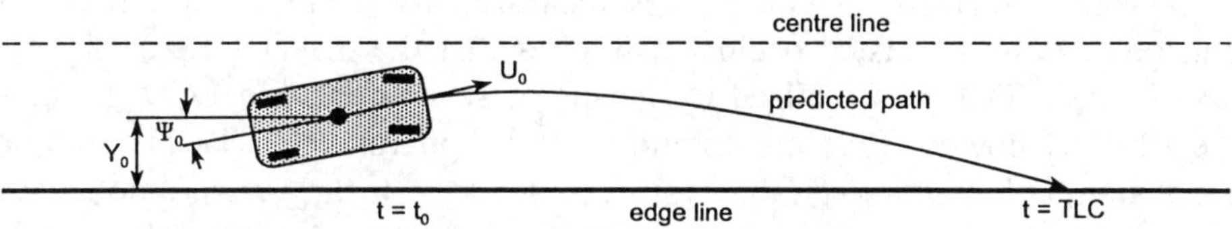

Figure 1 Schematic presentation of the path prediction in the TLC calculation.

2.1   Method

6 Subjects drove an instrumented vehicle on a 2 km straight track. The handling characteristics of the vehicle were varied by means of tyre pressure changes. Three pressure conditions of the tyres on the rear axle were included:
- 2.8 bar (standard tyre pressure for the instrumented car), giving normal understeer;
- 2.2 bar, resulting moderate understeer;
- 1.8 bar, resulting somewhat understeer.

Four different lane widths, 2.13, 2.63, 3.13, 3.63 m, were marked by cones on both sides together with a solid line on the left. Speed was kept constant at 100 km/h by means of a servo device.

System and driver performance data were registered, including lateral position, heading angle and steering angle. TLCs were calculated based on lateral position, heading angle, steering angle, the lane width and the width of the car. The steering wheel angle was evaluated in the frequency domain. A spectral density function of the steering wheel angle was calculated using a Fast-Fourier-Transformation. The amount of high frequency steering (HFS) was quantified as the ratio between the energy in the frequency band between 0.3 and 0.6 Hz and the energy in the frequency band between 0 and 0.6 Hz. A large HFS, usually due to a high frequency peak, is associated with difficult driving situations [1], [5].

The visual information demand was measured by means of a visual occlusion technique. Visual occlusion implies that the driver's field of view is obscured. This was realised by means of spectacles with LCD glasses, the PLATO device (Portable Liquid-crystal Apparatus for Tachistoscopic Occlusion) [6]. Only when drivers pressed a switch they were able to see the outside world for a short, preset period of time. An index for visual workload is derived by the average time after which drivers 'open' the PLATO glasses to look at the road in order to maintain a proper steering performance.

A prerequisite for the identification of valid vehicle handling predictors is reliability of the assessment. Based on an analysis of standards and scale design recommendations, a two level sequential judgement scale was designed with the following characteristics:
- Questions and instructions are integrated in the scale;
- Positive numbers are used as anchors;
- Verbal gradations are used at all anchors except for the terminal anchors;
- Bipolar scale is arranged symmetrically to the scale middle;
- Scale gradations are precise, in simple language, psychologically scaled and equally interspaced.
- The scale is organised in two levels requiring two assessments in sequence, the first being coarse and the second being a fine one. In this way choices are kept simple, while retaining the precision of a long scale.

An example of a Two-Level Sequential Judgement Scale for straight lane driving is given in Fig. 2.

In the experiment subjects started with two training runs, one at 60 km/h and one at 100 km/h. These were followed by four measuring runs, two without and two with occlusion. After completion of the runs for one tyre pressure*lane width combination, the driver was asked to rate steering difficulty. The sequence of tyre pressures and lane widths was randomised as far as possible. A detailed description of the experiment is given in [4].

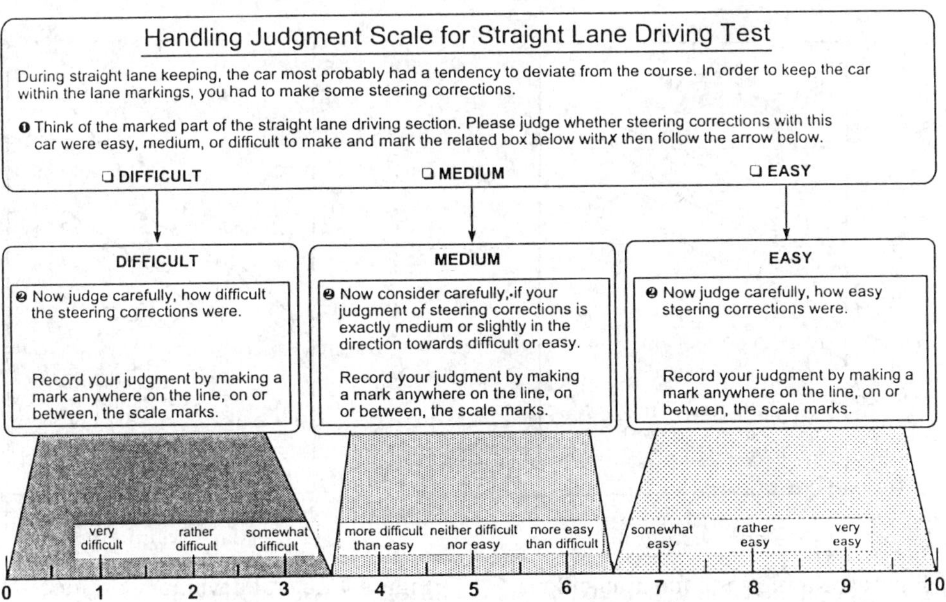

Figure 2 Two level sequential judgement scale for straight lane driving experiments

2.2   Results

Both lane width and tyre pressure had a main effect on assessments, as illustrated in Fig. 3. Assessment and tyre pressure ranks were identical and highest ratings resulted from highest rear pressure. The largest pressure effects were created at width 2.63 and 3.13 m.

The average lateral position varied with road width. Mean position was not in the middle of the lane, but shifted more to the left with wider lanes. No significant effect of tyre pressure on average lateral position was found. The standard deviation of the lateral position is regarded as an important system performance measure. The standard deviation of the lateral position as function of lane width for three tyre pressure conditions is illustrated in Fig. 4. Similar to the average lateral position an effect of lane width on the standard deviation was found. Deviations ranged from 0.05 m at lane width 2.13 m to 0.10 m at width 3.63 m. Again no effect of tyre pressure was found, indicating that drivers compensate for those differences.

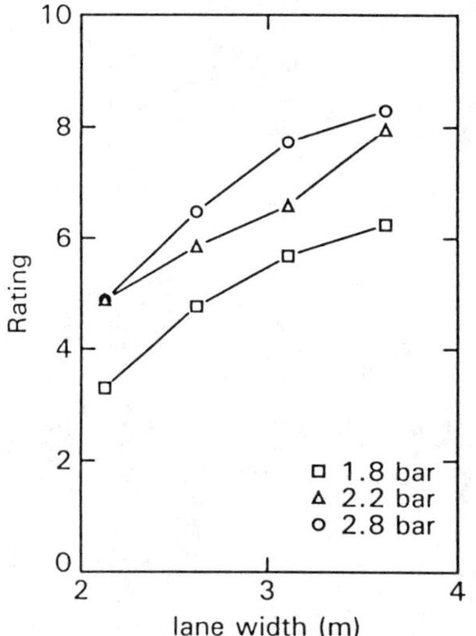

Figure 3 Ratings as a function of lane with for different tire pressure conditions

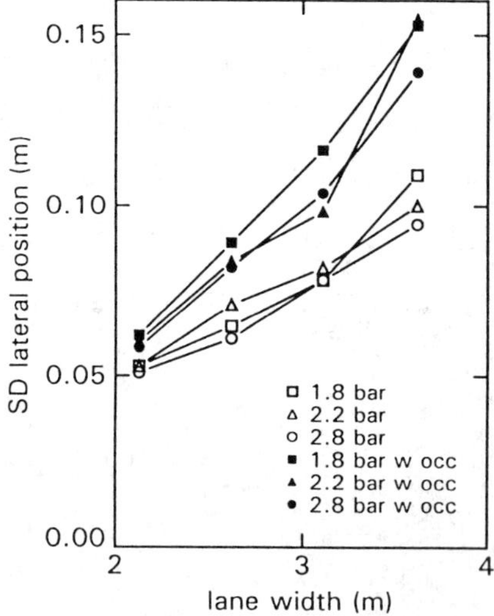

Figure 4 Lateral deviation as a function of lane width for different rear tire pressure without and with occlusion

Spectral density of the steering angle shows that high freq peaks appeared with increasing understeer as illustrated in Fig. 5. Fig. 6 shows the proportion of high frequency steering (HFS) which increased with decreasing tyre pressure (decreasing understeer). This confirms that drivers were able to keep their performance constant by increasing their steering effort in order to compensate for increased task difficulty. The effect of lane width on high fr equency steering did not show the same monotonous ranking as assessment did. A remarkable shift of steering energy to higher frequencies occurred at lane width 3.13 m.

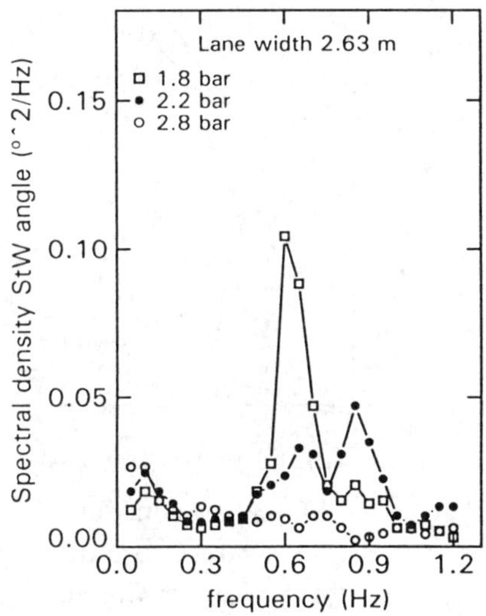

Figure 5   Spectral density of steering
            wheel angle for lane width
            2,63m for different tyre pres-
            sure without occlusion

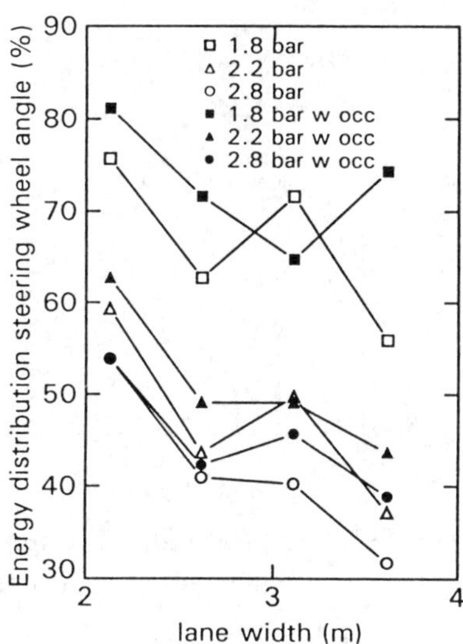

Figure 6   Proportion of high
            frequency steering (HFS)
            as a function of lane
            width for different tyre
            pressures without occlusion.

Average occlusion time is given in Fig. 7. Lane width had a significant effect, but tyre pressure did not. One conclusion is that driver adaptation to different handling qualities was successful by increase steering effort without requiring increasing driver input in terms of visual sampling rate.

Median TLC and the 15-percentile TLC showed identical characteristics. Fig. 8 illustrates the $TLC_{15\%}$. Both lane width and tyre pressure had a significant main effect, while also the ranking was monotonous just like the assessment ranking. Occlusion did not have a significant effect on TLC. The TLC at the end of the occlusion period, which is a measure for the margin remaining for error correction after a period of error neglection is indicated in Fig. 9, showing a similar characteristic as the 15-percentile TLC and the assessment scores.

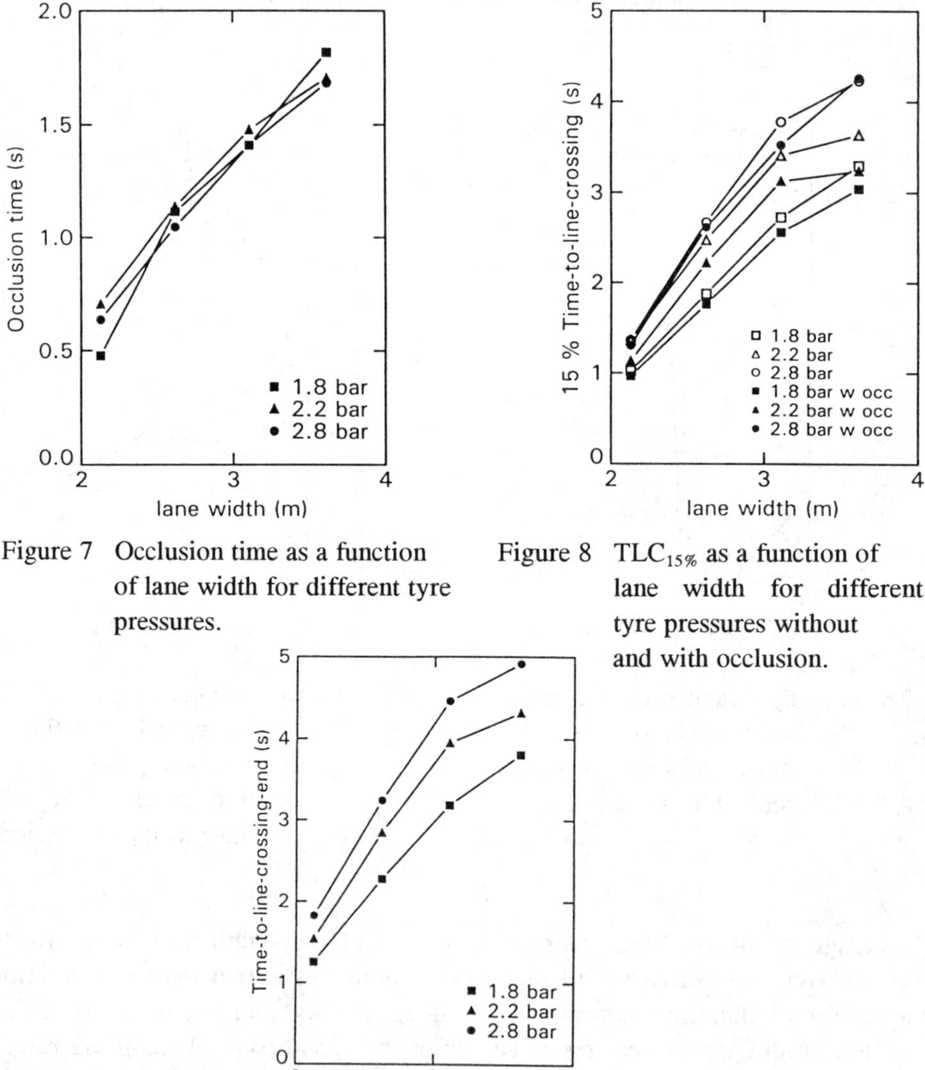

Figure 7   Occlusion time as a function of lane width for different tyre pressures.

Figure 8   TLC$_{15\%}$ as a function of lane width for different tyre pressures without and with occlusion.

Figure 9 TLC$_{end}$ as a function of lane width for different tyre pressures.

2.3   Discussion

The results show that Time to Line Crossing is a good predictor of the effect of both road characteristics and vehicle characteristics on assessment. Lateral performance only reflects the effect of road characteristics, while drivers compensate for deteriorated vehicle handling by means of increasing steering effort. Though steering effort is sensitive to handling variations it was found not to be a good predictor of the effect of lane width on assessment. Visual sampling in terms of occlusion time proved only to reflect the effect of lane width, but not the effect of handling variations on assessment.

As expected from the fact that TLC is an integrated measure of vehicle characteristics, driver steering and road characteristics, the prediction of car handling assessment by TLC had the highest quality. This finding was confirmed in a study of truck handling assessment [7].

3. DRIVER SUPPORT AND VISUAL WORKLOAD

Not only can the lateral control task be alleviated by improved vehicle handling characteristics, but also feedback on course deviations could be improved. A lane keeping support system, such as the Heading Control (HC) system developed by BMW, assists the driver by giving proprioceptive feedback via the steering wheel. Supporting the steering task may prevent drivers from running off the road or into an adjacent lane. In addition, it may also reduce the workload of keeping the vehicle on course. A Heading Control system provides a torque on the steering wheel to support the driver in the steering task, in case the vehicle deviates from a proper course. With this system drivers are kept in the control loop at all times, having full control of the vehicle. In a field experiment the effects of the Heading Control system on visual workload and steering behaviour were studied [12].

3.1   Method

The test vehicle used in the experiment was equipped with a prototype of a Heading Control system. The HC system detects the course of the road ahead by means of video image processing of the right or left lane markings. Based on the lateral position of the vehicle, its heading angle and the curvature of the road, the HC system calculates an optimal steering wheel angle. The error signal between optimal steering wheel angle and the actual steering wheel angle is translated into a proportional feedback torque that is generated by a torque motor on the steering column. The proprioceptive cue provided by the additional steering wheel torque indicates in what direction the steering wheel should be turned. The optimal steering wheel angle is determined by means of an optimal pre-view compensation algorithm with a pre-view of 0.6 s ahead of the vehicle [8].

Similar as in the vehicle handling experiment, visual workload was measured by means of occlusion.

Eight male subjects took part in the experiment on a motorway section, closed to other traffic. Runs were made at 80 and 120 km/h, in daylight and at night. Furthermore the lane width was varied on two levels: 2.75 m and 3.25 m. Half the runs were made with assistance of the HC systems, in the other half the HC system was switched off. Both runs without and with occlusion were made. All subjects drove all conditions twice. The order of conditions was counter balanced, except for light conditions. Subjects were instructed not to open the occlusion glasses more often than necessary to maintain a proper course and to stay within the lane boundaries.

The experiment was analyzed in terms of average occlusion time (T_{occ}), standard deviation of the lateral position, proportion of high frequency steering (HFS), minimum TLC (TLC_{min}) and the TLC at the end of the occlusion period (TLC_{end}). For each of the dependent variables an analysis of variance (ANOVA) was conducted with factors HC (on / off), Occlusion (without / with), Speed (80 / 120 km/h), Lane width (2.5 / 3.25 m) and Light (day / night).

3.2   Results

Heading Control was found to have a main effect on the average occlusion time. The occlusion time (T_{occ}) increased from 1.55 s (HC off) to 2.02 s when the HC-system was switched on [$F(1,7)=32.6$, $p<0.01$], indicating that HC reduces visual workload. Visual workload increased with increasing speed, decreasing lane width and at night. At night the occlusion time was shorter than in day light, i.e. 1.50 s versus 2.06 s [$F(1,7)=67.5$, $p<0.001$]. When the lane width was reduced from 3.25 m to 2.5 m T_{occ} reduced from 2.12 s to 1.45 s [$F(1,7)=54.8$, $p<0.001$].

Speed yielded a T_{occ} of 2.04 s at 80 km/h and 1.53 s at 120 km/h [F(1,7)=317, p<0.001].

All interactions between HC and the other factors were significant: HC x Light [F(1,7)=11.0, p<0.05], HC x Lane width [F(1,7)=11.8, p<0.05], HC x Speed [F(1,7)=9.3, p<0.05]. Additional post-hoc comparisons (Tukey-test) showed that both in daylight conditions (p<0.001) and in the dark (p<0.001) the occlusion time increased when the HC system was on. There was no significant difference between the nighttime condition with Heading Control and the daytime condition without Heading Control, indicating that the effect of HC is of the same order as the effect of light condition, see Figure 10. Also, in both speed conditions the occlusion time increased with the HC-system on (p<0.001), see Figure 11. Again there was no significant difference between the occlusion time with the HC-system at 120 km/h and without HC at 80 km/h, indicating that the effect of HC is comparable to the effect of a speed reduction of 40 km/h. The interaction between the HC system and lane width showed that in the wide lane condition there was a significant increase of the occlusion time when the HC-system was on (p<0.001). A Tukey test on the narrow lane condition showed no significant effect of HC on the occlusion time, see Figure 12. This suggests an increase of the effectiveness of HC with increasing lane width.

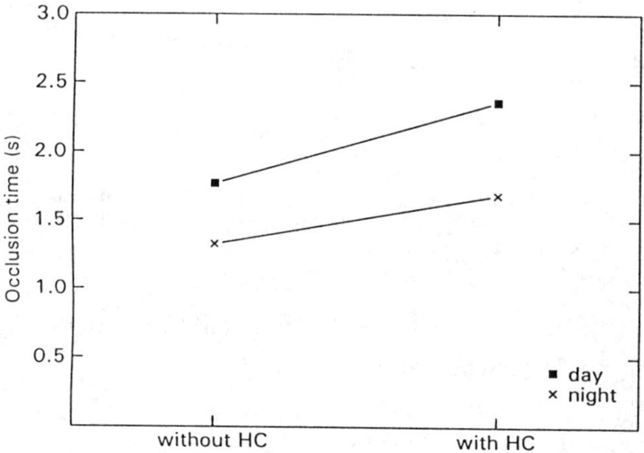

Figure 10   Occlusion time without and with Heading Control in day and night condition.

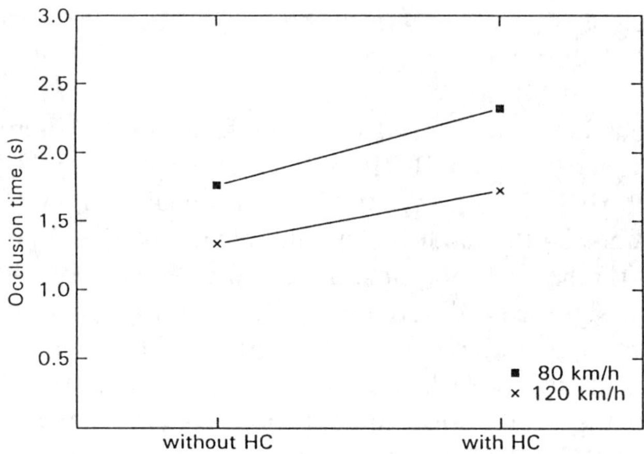

Figure 11   Occlusion time without and with Heading Control at 80 km/h and at 120 km/h.

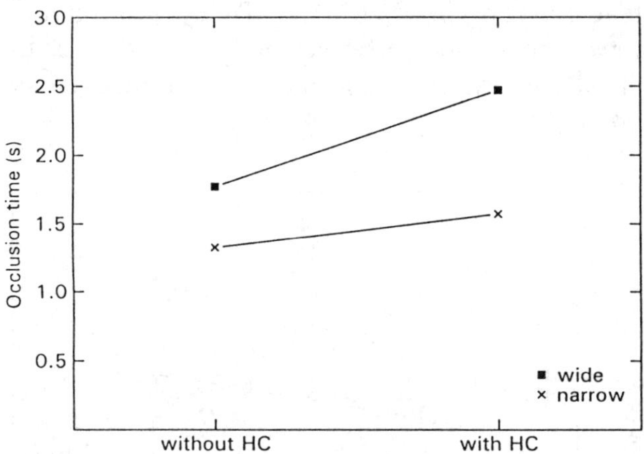

Figure 12   Occlusion time without and with Heading Control in narrow and wide lane condition.

Due to the HC system the standard deviation of the lateral position (SDLP) decreased from 0.16 m to 0.14 m [$F(1,7)=6.34$, $p<0.05$], suggesting that HC improved steering performance. With occlusion the SDLP increased from 0.13 m (no occlusion) to 0.18 m (with occlusion) [$F(1,7)=69.8$, $p<0.001$], which is a similar effect of occlusion on lane keeping performance as was found in the handling assessment experiment. The effect of Heading Control and occlusion on SDLP is illustrated in Figure

13. In the wide lane condition the SDLP was 0.17 m against 0.13 m in the narrow lane condition [$F(1,7)=77.2$, $p<0.001$]. Night time conditions resulted in a SDLP of 0.17 m versus 0.13 m in daylight [$F(1,7)=11.3$, $p<0.05$]. There was no significant effect of speed [$F(1,7)=0.75$, n.s.].

Comparison of the SDLP in the condition without occlusion to the effects found in a Heading Control experiment by Schumann et al. [8], shows that the course deviations in the visual workload experiment were in general smaller, but the effect of the HC system was larger. The SDLP in the Schumann experiment reduced by 6% from 0.32 m without HC to 0.3 m with a pre-view compensation HC strategy. Under comparable conditions in the visual workload experiment (no occlusion, daylight, normal lane width, 120 km/h) the SDLP was reduced by 18% from 0.13 m without HC to 0.11 m with HC.

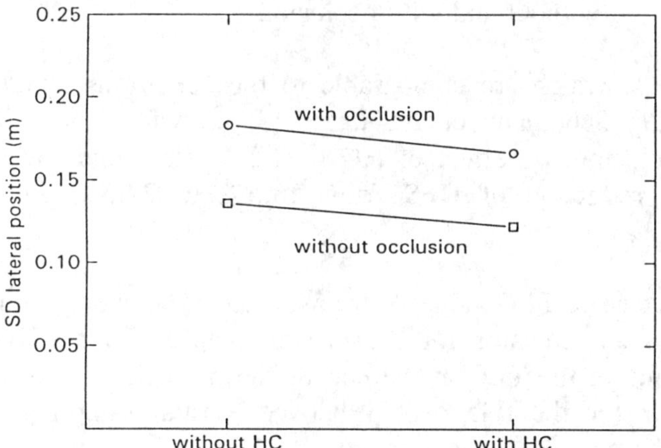

Figure 13   Standard deviation of the lateral position (SDLP) as a function of Heading Control

Heading Control reduced the proportion of high frequency steering (HFS) from 29.1% to 27.0% [$F(1,7)=6.18$, $p<0.05$]. Decreasing lane width causes an increase of the HFS from 26.1% in the wide lane condition to 30.1% in the narrow lane condition [$F(1,7)=20.8$, $p<0.01$]. An interaction between speed and HC was found [$F(1,7)=19.0$, $p<0.01$], indicating that HC mainly reduced the difficulty of steering in the 80 km/h condition. The interaction between light, occlusion and HC [$F(1,7)=18.8$, $p<0.01$] shows that in difficult conditions, i.e. at night, with occlusion, the effect of HC on HFS was most pronounced (see Figure 14).

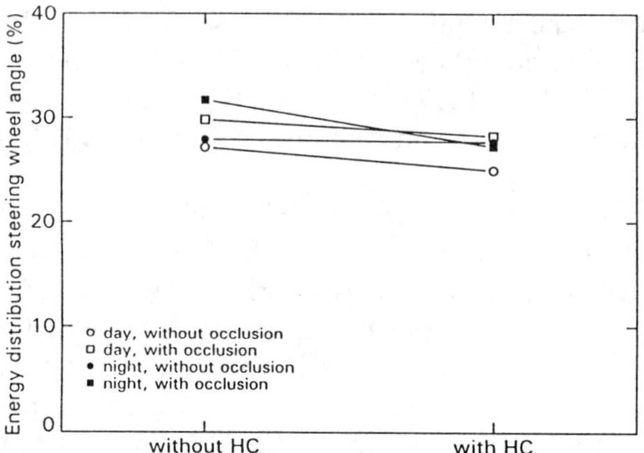

Figure 14   Proportion of high frequency steering (HFS) as a function
                   of Heading Control for day and night time conditions,
                   without and with occlusion.

In conditions, which are comparable to the conditions in the experiment
conducted by Schumann et al., i.e. daylight, wide lane, 120 km/h and
without occlusion, no effect of HC on HFS was found. Schumann et al.
reported a reduction of HFS from 26.5% to 22.5% due to Heading
Control.

Two characteristic TLC values were analyzed: The average minimum TLC
(TLC_{min}) as an indicator for the margin realised by the driver and the
average value of the TLC at the end of the occlusion periods (TLC_{end}) as
an indicator for the relationship between visual sampling strategy and
course deviations.

The minimum TLC increased as a consequence of the Heading Control
system from 3.49 s to 3.70 s [$F(1,7)=5.59$, $p<0.05$], indicating that HC
enabled subjects to increase their safety margin. Decreasing lane width
caused a reduction of the TLC_{min} from 4.11 s to 3.07 s [$F(1,7)=130$,
$p<0.001$]. The TLC_{min} was also reduced due to occlusion [$F(1,7)=13.1$,
$p<0.01$] and due to a speed increase [$F(1,7)=9.44$, $p<0.05$]. Light
condition had no significant effect on TLC_{min} [$F(1,7)=0.97$, n.s.].

Again the average TLC at the moment the PLATO glasses were opened,
TLC_{end}, reduced with increasing speed [$F(1,7)=60.3$, $p<0.001$] and with
decreasing lane width [$F(1,7)=56.3$, $p<0.001$]. Heading Control and

light condition had no significant main effect (respectively [$F(1,7)=0.4$, n.s.] and [$F(1,7)=0.39$, n.s.]).

TLC_{end} as found in the present experiment is larger than the values reported in the handling assessment experiment. As TLC_{end} proved to be strongly correlated to vehicle handling characteristics, this was to be expected. Apart from absolute differences, relative effects in the HC experiment are similar to other experiments. In an experiment by Godthelp (1984) the ratio of TLC_{end} at 80 km/h and TLC_{end} at 120 km/h was 1.28. In the handling experiment the ratio between TLC_{end} at a lane width of 3.25 m and at 2.5 m was 1.6. In the present experiment these ratios are respectively 1.33 and 1.46.

3.3   Discussion

When occlusion time is translated into visual workload, it can be concluded that Heading Control reduced visual workload. HC increased the average occlusion time from 1.55 s to 2.02 s (30.3% increase). In the baseline condition subjects looked at the road for 24.4% of the time, while with HC this percentage dropped to 19.8%. Even with less visual information the steering accuracy improved. The standard deviation of the lateral position was reduced from 0.183 m to 0.166 m (9.3% improvement). Based on a slight reduction of the high frequency component of steering behaviour, it can be concluded that the improved performance was not a result of increased steering effort but of improved quality of the steering control (no faster steering corrections but more appropriate corrections).

The increase of the TLC_{min} by Heading Control in all conditions shows that the safety margin that can be maintained has increased. The absence of an effect of HC control on the TLC at the moment the occlusion glasses are opened, indicates that HC does not influence the looking strategy. These findings indicate that the proprioceptive information from the HC system is not just used by the driver as a switching trigger between error neglection and error correction (this would only reduce visual workload, without an improvement of lateral performance), but it is actually integrated as a feedback loop in the steering control.

A detailed analysis (reported in [12]) of the effects of a sudden disturbance, introduced by a transition of transversal gradient of the test track, showed that the HC system helps drivers to compensate for such disturbances. When a driver is looking away from the road in the unsupported situation, an unexpected disturbance could lead to an unacceptable deviation. As Blaauw [1] showed, the driver will look at the road again when his internal prediction of the deviation (and its uncertainty) surpasses a certain threshold. Due to the disturbance the deviation may become larger than the prediction. In the supported situation the proprioceptive information provides the driver with an indication of the actual deviation which on the one hand reduces the uncertainty and on the other hand provides the cue to compensate for the disturbance.

In the experiment of Schumann et al. [8], comparing different HC algorithms, both an improvement of the lateral performance and a reduction of the steering effort was found for the pre-view compensation algorithm as used in the visual workload study. Under comparable conditions, that is without occlusion, daylight, 120 km/h and normal lane width, the visual workload study showed a reduction in course deviations, without an effect on the proportion of high frequency steering behaviour. The main difference between the two experiments was the task. In Schumann's experiment subjects performed multiple tasks as they drove on an open motorway, amongst other traffic, i.e. both lateral and longitudinal control, while probably also attention had to be given to higher tasks levels (not just the control level but also manoeuvre level, e.g. overtaking). The visual workload experiment focused on lateral control as a single control task. The effect of HC on lateral position, as found in this visual workload experiment, is larger than the effect found in the Schumann experiment (18% reduction of the standard deviation versus 6% in the Schumann experiment), while there is no effect on steering behaviour. The difference in absolute levels of standard deviation of the lateral position between the experiments, provides evidence for the notion that in the present experiment there was more emphasis on lateral performance than in the Schumann experiment. As noted in Schumann's experiment lateral control was just one of many tasks to be attended. The standard deviation in the present experiment was 50% of the standard deviation found by Schumann. It seems natural that when emphasis is put on one single task the effect of a support system is translated into an improvement of performance on that task rather than in a reduction of effort, while in a multi task situation the gain provided by a support system is partially translated in a reduction in effort to the benefit of other tasks.

In summary, Heading Control relieves visual workload and improves steering performance, especially under normal motorway conditions. In case of unexpected course disturbances, the Heading Control system provides valuable support.

4. SUBJECTIVE ASSESSMENT OF AUTOMATED DRIVING

A step further than supporting drivers while performing their task is to have an automated system performing that very task. Through the fast and accurate responses that an automated vehicle guidance (AVG) system is capable of, shorter margins could be realised, making more efficient use of the available asphalt. Short headways and tight steering would allow high traffic densities and narrow lanes, however in the end people will have to be prepared to make use of such a high performance transportation system. Moreover in case automated driving is possible on part of the road network, at some stage a manual control will have to be resumed. An automated system will have to provide a condition in which a driver is capable to safely and comfortably take over control. A series of driving simulator studies was performed to investigate what impact the main characteristics of an automated vehicle guidance system have on user acceptance. In a first study drivers were asked to give ratings on comfort in different headway conditions, while being driven on a highway with the left lane dedicated to automated travel [11]. A second study compared different levels of support during the transfer of control to the driver. It also looked at the impact of traffic conditions on the ease and safety of leaving an automated lane [10]. The study which is discussed in this paper focused on the acceptance of tight margins in lateral direction [9].

4.1   Method
The experiment was conducted in the TNO driving simulator. This is an interactive simulator, with a mock-up of a passenger car. Computer generated images were projected on a cylindrical screen with a horizontal visual angle of 120° [3].

In one part of the experiment the subjects drove in an automated mode on an automated lane with varying width, partly physically separated from the manual traffic lanes by means of a barrier and partly directly adjacent to the normal manual traffic lanes. In the other part of the experiment, subjects drove the same route while steering the car themselves.

The part in which subjects drove under automated control included the following conditions:

Lane width: 2.0, 2.75, 3.5 m
Physical separation: without barrier, with barrier
AVG speed: 80, 105, 130 km/h

In the manual runs only the lane configuration was varied:
Lane width: 2.0, 2.75, 3.5 m
Physical separation: without barrier, with barrier

By means of a button board, subjects gave a subjective rating about the driving situation. This box was mounted to the right side of the steering wheel at an easy reaching distance from the subject. There were seven buttons: three red ones on the left side, three geen ones on the right side and a half red / half green button in the middle. In this way a seven-point scale was established ranging from very uncomfortable to very comfortable.

In total 8 subjects participated in the simulator experiment. Both male and female subjects participated. Subjects were selected on the following criteria: age between 21 and 55 years, in the possession of a driving licence for more than 3 years and driving more than 10.000 km per year.

For the automated trial an analysis of variance (ANOVA) was performed on the comfort ratings with factors Lane width (2, 2.75, 3.5 m), Physical separation (without, with) and AVG-speed (80, 105, 130). For the manual trials ANOVAs with factors Lane width and Physical separation were performed on comfort rating, driving speed, average lateral position, standard deviation of the lateral position and on the proportion of high frequency steering.

4.2   Results

Only the factor lane width showed a main effect $[F(2,14)=21.0, p<0.001]$ on the comfort ratings in the automated trials. No significant effects of physical separation $[F(1,7)=0.11, \text{n.s.}]$ and speed $[F(2,14)=1.53, \text{n.s.}]$ were found. Fig. 15 shows the comfort rating as a function of lane width.

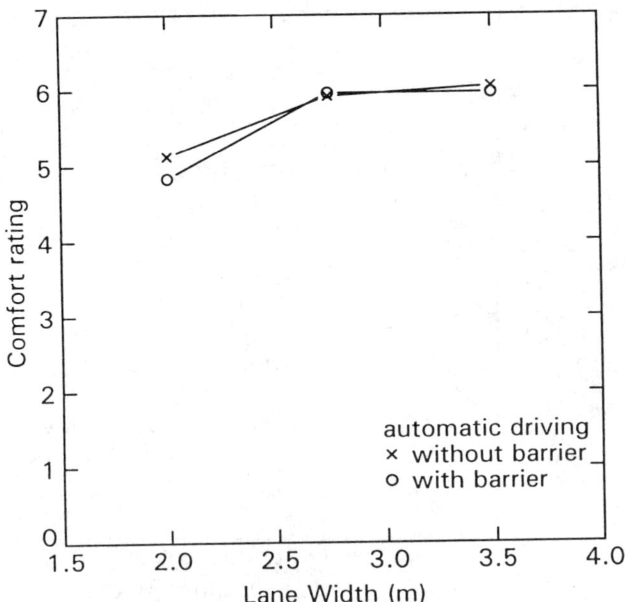

Figure 15   Comfort rating in the automated trails as a function of lane width, without and with barrier.

For the comfort separation [F(1,7)=11.1, p<0.05] and lane width [F(2,14)=27.4, p<0.001] ratings in the manual trials an effect of both physical was found. As illustrated in Fig. 16 similar to the automated mode comfort decreases with decreasing lane width, however in contrast to the automated mode the presence of a barrier reduces comfort while driving manually.

Main effects on driving speed were found of physical separation [F(1,7)=25.7, p<0.01] and lane width [F(2,14)=25.8, p<0.001]. The driving speed is adapted to the lane condition: subjects reduced their speed in narrow lanes and in the presence of a barrier (see Fig. 17). At the largest lane width without barrier average speed was 116 km/h, while in the most narrow lane with barrier average speed dropped to 78 km/h.

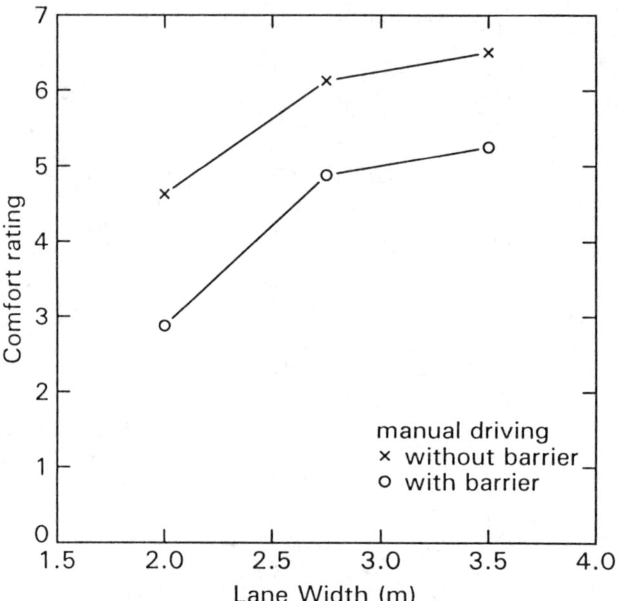

Figure 16   Comfort rating in the manual trails as a function of lane width, without and with barrier.

In this experiment no significant effect of lane width on average lateral position was found [$F(2,14)=0.04$, n.s.]. The presence of a barrier caused a shift of the average lateral position [$F(1,7)=1.47$, $p<0.01$] from 0.08 m to the left of the centre of the lane without barrier to 0.43 m left of the centre of the lane with barrier.

Standard deviation of the lateral position showed no main effect of physical separation [$F(1,7)=0.84$, n.s.]. There was a trend of decreasing standard deviation with decreasing lane width [$F(2,14)=3.18$, $p<0.1$]. Standard deviations ranged from 0.07 m. in the wide lane condition to 0.016 m. in the narrow lane condition with barrier, showing that subjects steered very accurately to stay within the narrow lane (Fig. 18). In coherence with this result it was found that the proportion of high frequency steering increased with decreasing lane width [$F(2,14)=6.56$, $p<0.01$], while this measure was not affected by physical separation [$F(1,7)=0.32$, n.s.].

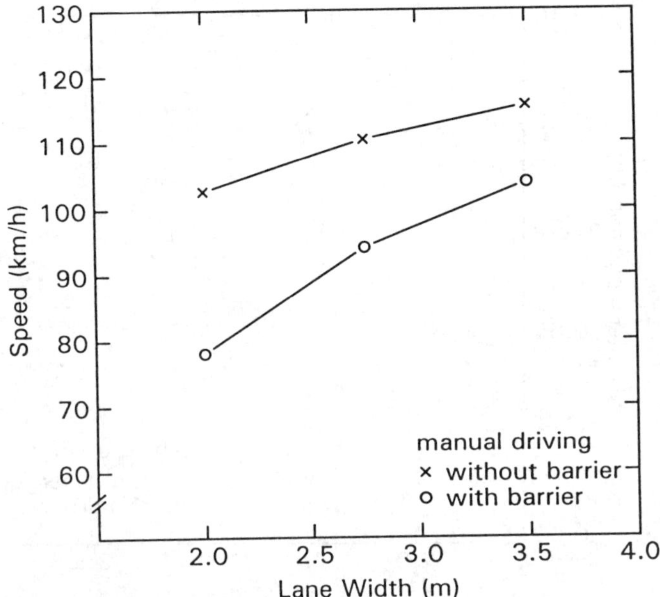

Figure 17   Driving speed in the manual trials as a function of lane width, without and with barrier.

4.3   Discussion

In order to cope with the narrow lane condition subjects reduced their speed and shifted their course away from the barrier. Steering effort was increased in the tight lane conditions, but not to a large extent, indicating that in a self paced situation adaptation is achieved through speed reduction. Given the design parameters of an automated lane, the present results provide a guideline for the maximum speed that should be respected before control of the vehicle is transferred from the autopilot to the driver. The presence of a barrier and driving speed are not a factor in the comfort of an AVG system. Therefore, a barrier between the automated lane and the manual lanes, installed for safety reasons, e.g. to prevent drivers in the manual lane from unintendedly entering the AVG lane, does not affect the acceptance of being driven in an AVG system. However a barrier is a discomfort factor in case of manual driving.

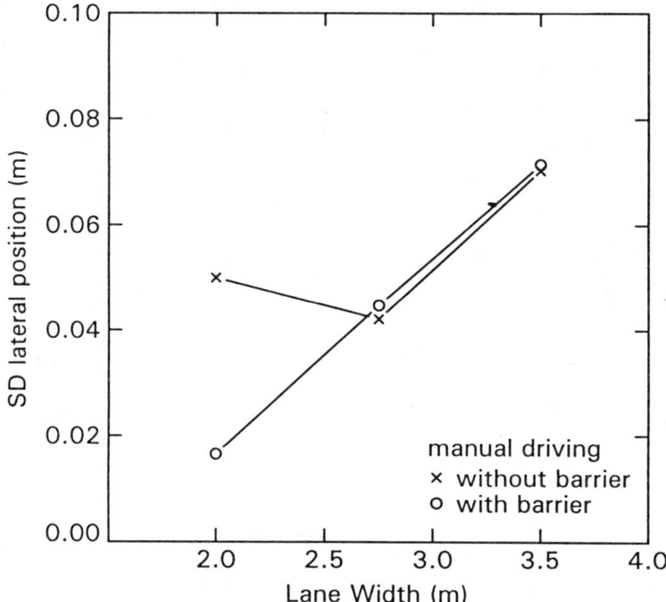

Figure 18   Standard deviation of the lateral position in the manual trials as a function of lane width, without and with barrier.

5. OVERALL DISCUSSION AND CONCLUSIONS

The results of the handling assessment study showed no effect of vehicle dynamics on the standard deviation of the lateral position nor on occlusion time. Tyre pressure was found to have an effect on high frequency steering, on TLC and on the subjective ratings. It seems that in the set-up of this tyre-pressure experiment, subjects compensated for the deterioration of handling characteristics by means of increased steering effort. In this way the steering performance remained unaffected by vehicle dynamics (Subjects received no specific lane-keeping instruction. The only instruction was to drive safely on a straight line. It was implied that subjects should not wander beyond the cones marking the lane). Handling characteristics did not affect visual workload. Although there is always the possibility of some trade off in steering strategy between performance, effort and visual workload it seems plausible that improved handling characteristics primarily reduce steering effort, while a lane keeping support system has the potential to relieve visual workload. In the first two experiments with fixed speed conditions, the adaptation to reduced lane margins was achieved through increased steering effort. In the last experiment with in the manual mode having the opportunity to adapt their speed subjects chose speed reduction over increasing steering effort to maintain the proper level of performance.

The overall conclusion can be that drivers adapt to the driving conditions. Depending on the task situation this adaptation is achieved through adaptation of effort as reflected by the proportion of high frequency steering or by adapting the visual sampling strategy or by adapting the task difficulty through speed adaptation. As drivers have these degrees of freedom to adapt to the driving conditions, just single measures of performance or steering do not suffice to predict assessment. By combining road characteristics and vehicle characteristics with driver strategy in terms of TLC, a measure reflecting driver assessment of handling characteristics can be achieved.

REFERENCES

[1]   Blaauw, G.J., *Car driving as a supervisory control task*. Dissertation TU Delft, TNO Institute for Perception, Soesterberg, 1984.

[2]   Godthelp, J., Milgram, P. & Blaauw, G.J., The development of a time-related measure to describe driving strategy. *Human Factors*, 26, pp. 257-268, 1988.

[3]   Hoekstra, W., van der Horst, R. & Kaptein, N.A., Visualisation of road design for assessing human factors aspects in a driving simulator. *Proceedings Driving Simulator Conference*, Lyon, France, 8-9 September, 1997.

[4]   Käppler, W.-D., Godthelp, J., *Design and use of the two-level sequential judgement scale in the identification of vehicle handling criteria: I. Instrumented car experiments on straight lane driving.* Report FAT 79, Forschungsinstitut für Anthropotechnik, Wachtberg, also Report IZF 1990 B-13, TNO Institute for Perception, Soesterberg, 1989.

[5]   McLean, J.R. & Hoffmann, R. (1975). Steering reversals as a measure of driver performance and steering task difficulty. *Human Factors*, 17(3), pp. 248-256, 1975.

[6]   Milgram, P., A spectacle-mounted liquid-crystal tachistoscope. *Behaviour Research Methods, Instruments, & Computers,* 19 (5), pp. 449-456, 1987.

[7]   Randwijk, M.J. van, Godthelp, J., Käppler, W.D. & Ruys, P.A.J., Correlation of driver judgements and vehicle directional data to evaluate and predict truck handling. *European Automobile Engineers Cooperation, EAEC paper No. 91054*, pp. 530-539, Strasbourg, 1991.

[8]   Schumann, J. Löwenau, J. & Naab, K., The active steering wheel as a continuous support for the driver's lateral control task. In: Gale, A.G. *Vision in Vehicles V* Elsevier, Amsterdam, 1996.

[9]   Vos, A.P. de, *Behavioural aspects of automated vehicle guidance (AVG); Lane width and Physical Separation.* TNO Human Factors Research Institute, Soesterberg, in preparation.

[10]   Vos, A.P. de, Hoekstra, W., Hogema, J.H., Soeteman, J.J., Acceptance of Automated Vehicle Guidance (AVG): System Reliability and Exit Manoeuvres. *Proceedings of the 4th World Congress on Intelligent Transport Systems*, Berlin, 1997.

[11]   Vos, A.P. de, Theeuwes, J., Hoekstra, W. & Coëmet, M.J., *Behavioral Aspects of Automated Vehicle Guidance (AVG); The Relationship between Headway and Driver Comfort.* Presented at TRB Annual Meeting, Washington, 12-16 January 1997.

[12]   Vos, A.P. de, J. Godthelp, J. Theeuwes & W.B. Verwey, *The influence of a Heading Control system on driver workload.* TNO report TM-96-C048, TNO Human Factors Research Institute, Soesterberg, 1996.

Vehicle Handling and Sensitivity in Transient Manoeuvres

Arvin. R. Savkoor, Hugo Happel, François Horkay

The subject of this paper is the dynamics of transient handling manoeuvres of vehicles controlled by human drivers. The paper addresses various issues of vehicle handling and the question of what constitutes good handling. The main discussion concentrates mainly on two distinct aspects. The first aspect analyses the driver's tasks of information processing and taking decisions concerning the appropriate control strategy (feed-forward and feedback) in response to different driving (environmental) situations The decisions taken by the human driver in actual steering and in the application of longitudinal control forces are based on two distinct types of information: 1) his/her internal working model of the inverse dynamics of the vehicle and 2) his/her ability to monitor, assess and process a large number of complex sets of cue (approaching road geometry, wind and weather conditions, traffic situation and the observed dynamic states of the vehicle). In view of the complexity and urgency of the driver's task it is argued that the driver's mental model of the inverse dynamics of the vehicle in transient manoeuvres is based on the simplest and most basic dynamic states of a vehicle that are consistent with his/her observations.

The second aspect of handling treated in this paper concerns a dynamic analysis of basic responses of a vehicle to steering input. The analysis using the simple 3 dof handling model may serve a vehicle designer as a preliminary design tool for gaining insight into the basic dynamic behaviour of a design. Another use of the simple analysis not elaborated in this paper is in the represention of the driver's inverse dynamic model for estimating control inputs according to the prospective vehicle path decision of the driver. The analysis considers the sensitivity of transient response of vehicles to changes in the design parameters of vehicles. A method of constructing sensitivity functions based on the response variables such as yaw rate, side-slip and roll angle is described..

1. INTRODUCTION

Most situations of driving involve transient lateral dynamics of vehicles. This fact implies that vehicle handling in transient manoeuvres is an important consideration in the preliminary design of road vehicles. A comprehensive evaluation and judgement of the handling performance is possible only by road-testing the prototype of a vehicle. Such testing implies the subjective involvement of driving the vehicle in the closed loop system consisting of the vehicle, the human driver and the real world environment. However because the iterative process of design and development of vehicles proves to be a time consuming and costly, it is necessary to consider the handling performance of the vehicle right from the start during the initial design phase of the vehicle. It is therefore desirable to build in the targeted handling qualities during the preliminary design of a vehicle. The goal in this initial design phase is to design the vehicle such that the handling performance of the vehicle + driver as a closed loop system approaches closely that targeted by the vehicle designer. Clearly, the target for the handling characteristics of vehicles may vary considerably depending upon the particular category of vehicles. The handling qualities expected by drivers in a given category depend strongly on the general driving performance (acceleration and top speed) and the expected degree of comfort. In the present paper the discussion is mainly restricted to ordinary, mass produced medium size passenger cars with adequate driving and handling performance.

The requirement for the handling behaviour of a vehicle depends upon the driving situation. The driving situations may be broadly divided into three categories:

1) Normal driving under favourable weather and light traffic conditions and   2) Driving under adverse weather and dense traffic conditions and

3) Critical situations demanded by an emergency.

The first situation is probably what a driver desires ideally in the sense that he or she usually appreciates a vehicle that is " fun to drive". The accent in the driving style is generally on vehicle performance related to acceleration, top speed and handling and/or a high degree of comfort.

The second situation arises under less favourable weather conditions that is when the visibility and the available friction are degraded and external forces due to side winds act on the vehicle. The driver has considerable difficulties in controlling the lateral, longitudinal and yaw motions of the vehicle. More often than not these conditions prompt a dramatic change in the style of driving, from the habitual style where control priority is on vehicle performance and comfort to a more defensive style oriented towards safety. On low friction (μ) surfaces and poor visibility conditions the vehicle dynamics tends to become strongly non-linear and the driver's view estimates of the road curvature become poorer. Under such conditions an average driver may find him/herself short of the lead time and experience to work out the inverse dynamics of the vehicle. As the feed-forward control becomes difficult to manage, the driver has to greatly increase his/her dependence on feedback control.

Unlike the second situation where the driver involvement is continuous for a significant period of time, the third situation occurs in the form of an "incident". The severe limitation on time puts a heavy demand on the information processing and decision taking abilities of the driver. At the same time the driver may be required to estimate and apply control inputs in situations where the vehicle dynamic behaviour becomes uncertain and non-linear. The application of large tangential forces (approaching the friction limit) and significant variations both in the available friction and vehicle speed lead to serious errors in the driver's inverse dynamic model and estimated inputs.

There is a strong case to use control devices for enhancing the stability and steerability of vehicles under emergency situations. The ABS, direct yaw moment control and 4 wheel steering are helpful provided the available tyre/road friction is sufficient (The recent lively interest in on-line μ estimation).

2. HANDLING IN THE DRIVER-VEHICLE-ENVIRONMENT SYSTEM

The study of handling requires mathematical models of the vehicle, the driver and the interaction of both the vehicle and the driver with the road and traffic environment. Vehicle dynamics modelling, although complex and laborious in detail , is conceptually straight forward to implement. Powerful and large scale multibody modelling programmes are generally available for modelling vehicles and calculating their dynamic response in great details. The practical limitation is the availability of reliable data of all the required parameters of the model. In contrast the greatest challenge in modelling is that concerning the information processing, decision making and action taking by the human driver.

The performance of the driver-vehicle system is intimately linked with the decisions and actions taken by the driver while driving the vehicle. The decisions and actions are based on two distinct types of information:

1) The drivers' mental working model of vehicle's dynamic behaviour

2) The drivers' ability to monitor, assess and process complex sets of cues (approaching road geometry, wind and weather conditions, traffic situation and the observed dynamic states of the vehicle).

Many driver models proposed in the open.literature consider the information and action of the driver as a form of preview tracking control (e.g. see [1]). In this volume Sharp [2] outlines a driver model for gathering sampled information of the path and the control strategy of the driver based on the optimal linear quadratic preview control.

Fuzzy logic and neural network methods are interesting developments for use in modelling systems involving complex physics because these methods develop establish the mathematical relationship between the relevant inputs and outputs without requiring any detailed knowledge of the physics of the system in question. In that sense The methodology makes use of empirical information ("training and experience") in a way similar to the operation of an average human driver. Kageyama and Pacejka [3] introduced a driver model that converts the visual information into a perceived risk level within the framework of a risk dependent fuzzy control model for driving The fuzzy control theory has been applied by Gu Xi and Yu Qun [4] to study handling and stability in transient manoeuvres of a closed loop driver-vehicle-environment system. Recently Yoshimoto et al, [5] presented a driver's course tracking model using dynamic visual information characterised by an optical flow of images.

The driver-vehicle interaction of information processing and control action is depicted in Figure 1.

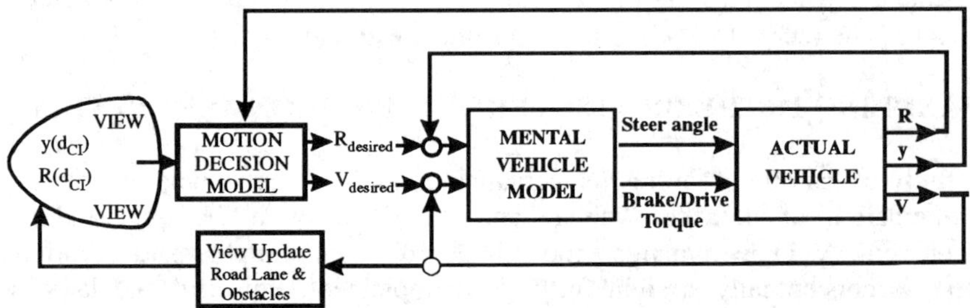

HUMAN DRIVER'S INFORMATION PROCESSING, MENTAL MODEL & CONTROL ACTION

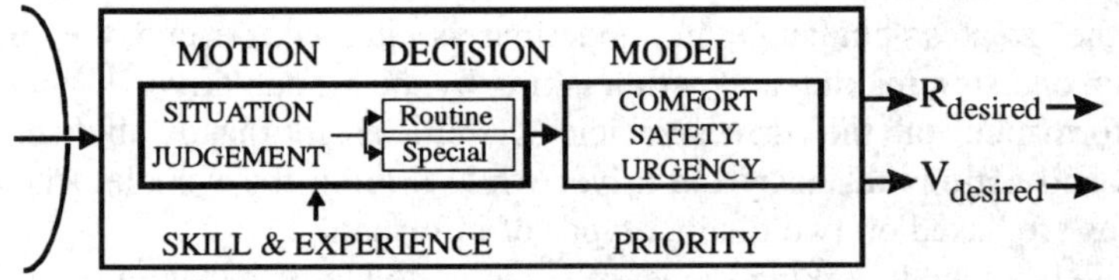

DETAILS OF THE MOTION DECISION PROCESS

Figure 1: The driver-vehicle interaction.

Clearly the complex tasks performed by the human driver raise the following questions:

- Can the driver cope up with this overload of information?
- Is the driver able to take split second decisions- the right decisions concerning the desired course of the vehicle in order to avoid obstacles and stick to the stipulated road lane (as far as possible)?
- Can the driver mentally work out the inverse dynamics of the vehicle and estimate the available control inputs (steer and brake or accelerate) which make the vehicle follow the desired course?

In a well-organised society there are many guidelines available to the driver concerning what the vehicle speed should be along the road lane that he or she is driving. The guidelines for the road builders and traffic authorities actually take into consideration the comfort and safety of the road user. The guidelines are based on a vehicle with an acceptable handling performance. Due consideration is given to shape the road geometry within the globally planned infrastructure and to the compatibility of the surfacing materials with the design speed under some average weather conditions and traffic situations expected locally. Often there are warning or advisory signs posted along the roads. The roads that are built and maintained by the road and transportation regulatory bodies already take into account the steering and braking requirements of vehicles. Their aim is to design roads which optimise the vehicle speed at which a human driver can travel with adequate comfort and safety under constraints imposed by the infrastructure, traffic and the environment.

The road design curvature and cant are actually based on the lateral dynamic behaviour of vehicles. For instance according to the guidelines in Gemini (RAS) of Forschungsgesellschaft für Straßen- und Verkehrswesen (Köln 1984).

The required lateral force coefficient for generating the centripetal acceleration of the vehicle travelling at a speed V along a curved road with radius of curvature ρ and cant gradient ζ is:

$$f_y \approx \frac{V^2}{\rho g} - \zeta \tag{1}$$

and the maximum lateral force coefficient (friction) for designing road curvature and camber is following Mitschke [6]:

$$\mu_{y\,max} = 0.198\,(V_d/100)^2 - 0.592(V_d/100) + 0.569 \tag{2}$$

where V_d is the desired design speed of the vehicle in km/h.

The utility factor ($f_y / \mu_{y\,max}$) depends upon the qualities of different types of roads for the corresponding ranges of allowable speeds.

One of the most important requirement of medium size passenger cars vehicles is a high degree of driving comfort both under normal and adverse weather driving conditions. In most cases the vehicle speed during handling manoeuvres is usually restricted in order to limit the lateral accelerations values not exceeding 0.3g. Interestingly, this is also a useful limit of lateral acceleration (on roads with μ of the order of unity) within which a linear analysis of vehicle lateral dynamics remains approximately valid.

Various test procedures (e.g. ISO standards) have been developed to evaluate handling of vehicles through subjective assessment by different categories of drivers including highly skilled test drivers. Certain (often unpleasant) aspects of dynamic behaviour of vehicles are inherently linked with objective factors of the intrinsic design of vehicles. While such aspects are minimised in well designed vehicles it is not always possible to assess their significance objectively in the initial design phase. In addition there is still no established method to quantify the threshold of human tolerance to complex and multiple dynamic disturbances. In such cases the vehicle manufacturer has to carry out subjective testing and assessment. The aim of the different tests carried out by vehicle manufacturers are intended to highlight a particular kind of dynamic behaviour and isolate the role played by any specific vehicle components or the design feature of the vehicle. An illustration of the standard handling manoeuvres used in field tests and computation has been presented by Loos and Dödlbacher [7].

The driver's overall evaluation of the handling quality of a vehicle is generally a weighted sum of partial evaluations of the different dynamic aspects of driving. In the present volume, Sharp [2] presents a clear and concise statement of how such aspects arise due to the specific design features of vehicles and the various test procedures for the subjective evaluation by the human driver.

A detailed analysis of subjective human judgement of the objective vehicle response using good driver models merits further investigations specially noting the differences in judgements between drivers with varying degrees of skill ranging from an average driver to a professional test driver. With an ever increasing level of performance and sophistication of modern vehicles it is but natural to demand an even quicker and more predictable response of vehicles to the control inputs applied by the driver. The desired vehicle characteristics for good handling are the same with all human operated vehicles irrespective of whether the vehicle uses conventional steering or some advanced control technology such as a 4 wheel steering, ABS, ASR and VDC.

The Criteria for Good Handling of Vehicles:

The desirable characteristics may be summarised as follows:

1) Shorter time delay (phase lag) in the yaw rate and lateral acceleration responses of the vehicle to steering input [Amongst others, Furukawa et al. [8].]. Loos and Dödlbacher [7] identify an optimum sub-region within the Weir / Di Marco region in the plot for the yaw velocity gain against the equivalent delay time. The gain is some measure of "the amount of reaction" while the peak response factor .T r_{max} (see Figure 6) is associated with the notion "quickness of response".

2) Good compromise between the requirements of sufficiently high damping of yaw rate and margin of stability on the one hand, and on the other hand the responsiveness of the vehicle to steering input.

3) Reduction of the body side-slip angle (off-tracking) [9] and keeping its magnitude and sign consistent with the driver's view requirements along the oncoming road lane [Objective with strong support but with some differences in details].

4) Increasing response immunity to external disturbances (crosswind, vertical and longitudinal excitations and road camber changes caused by uneven road surface) [Design objective with unanimous approval].

5) Reduction of the variation in the steering response with increasing vehicle speed and that due to the application of longitudinal forces of acceleration and braking [Well-recognised design objective].

6) Increasing robustness of driver-vehicle-environment system to moderate variations of vehicle, tyre parameters and the tyre/road friction [Design objective with unanimous approval].

7) Reducing the roll response [Objective with qualified approval]. Information feedback from the rolling motion has been studied by Nakagawa et al. [10].

8) Consistent feedback of information (steering torque, acceleration, roll and yaw) to the driver without significant reduction of comfort.
The information concerning the dynamic state and behaviour of the vehicle is transmitted to the driver through the driver-vehicle mechanical interface (steering wheel, seat, pedals etc). Any disinformation or inconsistency in the signals should be minimised and discomfort reduced {Well understood objective but one requiring more detailed investigation].

9) Signalling and warning the driver of any strong non-linearity as the tyre to road friction approaches the point of saturation without producing uncontrollable and unpredictable (to the inexperienced driver) responses from the vehicle [More recently emphasised research objective related to the problem of identification of tyre/road friction [11]].

Some of these requirements concerning the open loop vehicle dynamics are fairly obvious and universal. The open loop stability is unquestionably desirable; although the driver may be able to stabilise an inherently unstable vehicle to a certain extent the driver work load may induce fatigue or reduced concentration on other driving tasks. Similarly, there is little to quarrel about increasing immunity from external disturbances and requirements of consistent and robust open loop dynamics of vehicles.

Vehicle dynamic characteristics with respect to stability and responsiveness of yaw motion require some form of compromise based on the driver's subjective judgement. The requirement of an "ideal side slip angle" of the vehicle during transient manoeuvres requires more detailed examination of subjective road tests. Finally, the question that has to be answered is what should be the desired weighting factors on the different aspects of handling to achieve a good compromise between handling agility, stability (safety) and comfort expected from the particular class of drivers in the segment of the market for the vehicle.

Probably the second most difficult issue is the desired balance between the visual and non-visual (mechanical) information feedback and the compromise between feedback information and comfort. Clearly, the driver's subjective judgement is the deciding factor in this case.

The dynamic analysis of the handling response using a vehicle model in the early design stage enables the vehicle designer to assess the handling potential of a particular design and to choose appropriate values for the different vehicle parameters. The simulated response variables for various steering inputs may be translated into relevant objective characteristics of handling qualities of the vehicle. It is assumed that the subjective human judgement of handling quality may be correlated with certain objective characteristics of the vehicle.

From the discussion in the previous section it follows that the complexity and urgency of the driver's task demand that the driver's internal working model of vehicle dynamics be based on the simplest and most basic dynamic states of a vehicle that are consistent with his/her observations.

3.VEHICLE MODEL AND EQUATIONS OF MOTION

The vehicle model and the dynamic analysis in this paper is based on the following assumptions:
The driver's source of information concerning the vehicle dynamic behaviour is derived from the basic vehicle response which is represented by the lateral, yaw and roll motion of the vehicle The essential features of dynamic response of passenger cars to steering input can be described by a simple 3 dof bicycle model with two wheels with its centre of mass (gravity) located at some finite height above the road plane.
Undoubtedly the steering sub-system plays an important role in the subjective assessment of handling. The feel at the hand wheel and the dynamics of the steering gear are considered by some to be important criteria of handling qualities of vehicles. The steering torque felt by a driver gives useful information concerning the current state of the road wheels and friction. The steering gear ratio is chosen appropriately to reduce the effort and time required to turn the road wheels. However, ignoring the dynamics of the steering subsystem and the road wheels (possibility of shimmy, steering vibrations and the non-linear effects of backlash and dry friction for small steering angles) the major factor affecting subjective judgement is that concerned mainly with the ergonomic design of the subsystem and the vehicle.

The bicycle model of a four wheel vehicle with rigid body dynamics restricted to 3 degrees of freedom is shown in the figure 2. For simplicity, the steering system dynamics will not be considered in this paper. The pitch and bounce body-motions are ignored and the rolling motion of the body is assumed to take place by rotation about a roll axis located below the x-axis of a Cartesian co-ordinate frame (x,y,z) attached to the centre of gravity of the vehicle as shown in Figure. 2.
The equations of motion are developed in a co-ordinate frame fixed to the centre of gravity of the vehicle.

$$mV(\dot{\beta}+r) = F_{y1} + F_{y2}$$

$$I_x\dot{p} - I_{xz}\dot{r} + kp + c\varphi = h_1F_{y1} + h_2F_{y2} \tag{3}$$

$$I_z\dot{r} - I_{xz}\dot{p} = aF_{y1} - bF_{y2}$$

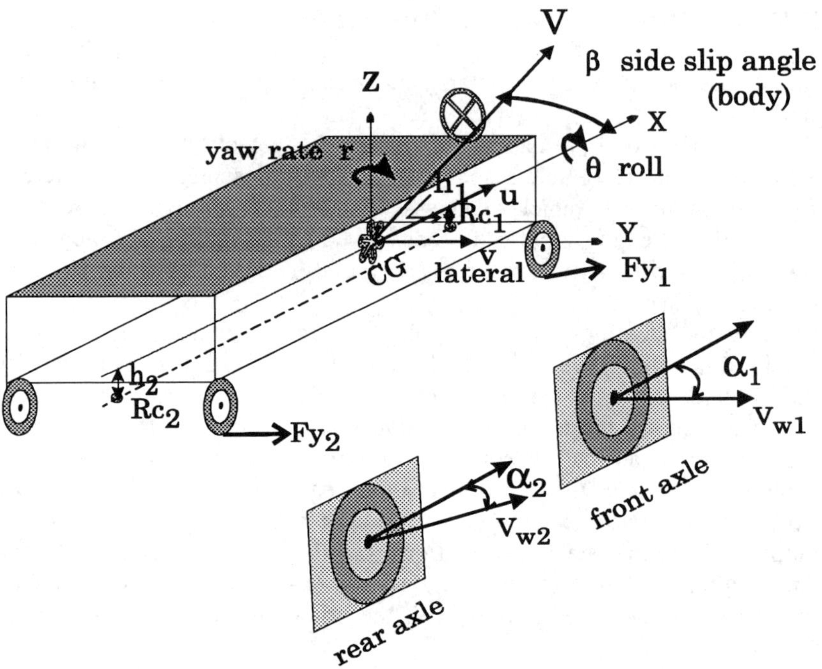

Figure 2: The vehicle (bicycle) model with a 3 dof body motion (lateral, yaw and roll) and two axles (the front (1) and rear (2)) showing the motion and forces acting on the body and the wheels.

Ignoring aerodynamic forces the most important external forces acting on the vehicle are the forces generated in the tyre/road contact. The lateral contact forces F_{y1} and F_{y2} generated by the front and rear tyres are functions of the respective slip angles, camber angle and the normal and longitudinal contact forces between the tyres and the road. Assuming constant normal loads, and small slip and camber angles and a road surface with high friction (coefficient), the lateral forces for stationary rolling with slip and camber are approximately linear functions of slip and camber angles.

$$F_{yi} = -C_i\,\alpha_i + C_{\gamma i}\,\gamma_i \; ; \quad i = 1,2. \tag{4}$$

where α and γ are the slip and camber angles and index $i = 1, 2$ refer to the variables of the front and rear axles respectively. The parameters C_i and $C_{\gamma i}$ are respectively the cornering and camber stiffness (the initial slopes of the linear tyre characteristics for $\alpha \to 0$ and $\gamma \to 0$).

$$-C_i = \left.\frac{\partial F_{yi}(\alpha_i)}{\partial \alpha_i}\right|_{\alpha_i=0,\gamma_i=0} \quad \text{and} \quad -C\gamma_i = \left.\frac{\partial F_{yi}(\gamma_i)}{\partial \gamma_i}\right|_{\alpha_i=0,\gamma_i=0} \tag{5}$$

The influence of elasto-kinematics of the vehicle suspension introduces coupling terms in camber and steering angle variations induced by the roll angle of the body and lateral forces. For small roll angles this influence may be taken into account in a linear approximation by introducing a roll-camber coupling parameter τ_i and a roll-steer coefficient ε_i .

The linearised equations for defining the kinematics including the suspension coupling effects read

$$\alpha_1 = \beta + \frac{a}{V}r + \frac{h_1}{V}p - \varepsilon_1\varphi - \delta; \quad \gamma_1 = \tau_1\varphi$$

$$\alpha_2 = \beta - \frac{b}{V}r + \frac{h_2}{V}p - \varepsilon_2\varphi; \quad \gamma_2 = \tau_2\varphi \tag{6}$$

The influence of non-stationary slip-rolling on the lateral tyre forces is introduced through a simple first order differential equation which describes the relaxation phenomenon of a tyre in terms of a relaxation length σ_i (a distance constant).

$$\frac{\sigma_i}{V}\dot{F}_{yi} + F_{yi} = \overset{*}{F}_{yi} \tag{7}$$

The tyre forces are then related to the vehicle motion through the following equations:

$$\frac{\sigma_1}{V}\dot{F}_{y1} + F_{y1} = -C_1\left\{\beta + \frac{a}{V}r + \frac{h_1}{V}p - \varepsilon_1\varphi - \delta\right\} + \tau_1 C_{\gamma 1}\varphi$$

$$\frac{\sigma_2}{V}\dot{F}_{y2} + F_{y2} = -C_2\left\{\beta - \frac{b}{V}r + \frac{h_2}{V}p - \varepsilon_2\varphi\right\} + \tau_2 C_{\gamma 2}\varphi \tag{8}$$

Upon introduction of the expression for the non-stationary tyre forces in equation (3) the equations of motion finally read:

$$mV(\dot{\beta}+r) = F_{y1} + F_{y2}$$

$$I_x\dot{p} - I_{xz}\dot{r} + kp + c\varphi = h_1 F_{y1} + h_2 F_{y2}$$

$$I_z\dot{r} - I_{xz}\dot{p} = aF_{y1} - bF_{y2} \qquad (9)$$

$$\frac{\sigma_1}{V}\dot{F}_{y1} + F_{y1} = -C_1\left\{\beta + \frac{a}{V}r + \frac{h_1}{V}p - \varepsilon_1\varphi - \delta\right\} + \tau_1 C_{\gamma 1}\varphi$$

$$\frac{\sigma_2}{V}\dot{F}_{y2} + F_{y2} = -C_2\left\{\beta - \frac{b}{V}r + \frac{h_2}{V}p - \varepsilon_2\varphi\right\} + \tau_2 C_{\gamma 2}\varphi$$

The equations of motion have been cast in the standard state space format

$$\dot{\overline{x}} = A\overline{x} + B\overline{u}$$

$$\overline{y} = C\overline{x} + D\overline{u} \qquad (10)$$

where the state vector x, the steering control input u and the output vector y are:

$$\overline{x}^T = \left| \beta \quad r \quad p \quad \varphi \quad F_{y1} \quad F_{y2} \right|$$

$$\overline{u} = \delta \qquad (11)$$

$$\overline{y}^T = \left| \beta \quad r \quad p \quad \varphi \right|$$

The matrices A, B , C and D are given in the appendix.

Response and parameter sensitivity in the frequency domain

The eigenfrequencies and the relative damping of the linear system as well as the frequency response functions of the vehicle motion variables to steering inputs have been calculated. Some typical results for the gains of transfer functions of lateral acceleration, slip rate, yaw rate and the roll rate are shown in Figure 3.
The influence of changes in the values of some of the relevant parameters on the magnitude of the frequency response functions can be seen in Figures 4 and 5. The influence of varying the cornering stiffness of tires on the lateral and yaw motions is, as expected, significant. The rolling motion, on the other hand, depends strongly on the moment of inertia about the longitudinal axis, the height of the centre of gravity and the suspension roll stiffness and damping. The frequency response functions are less suited to reveal subtle differences in the transient response of vehicles due to small variations in the vehicle parameters. The transient response is well represented in the time domain which will be considered next

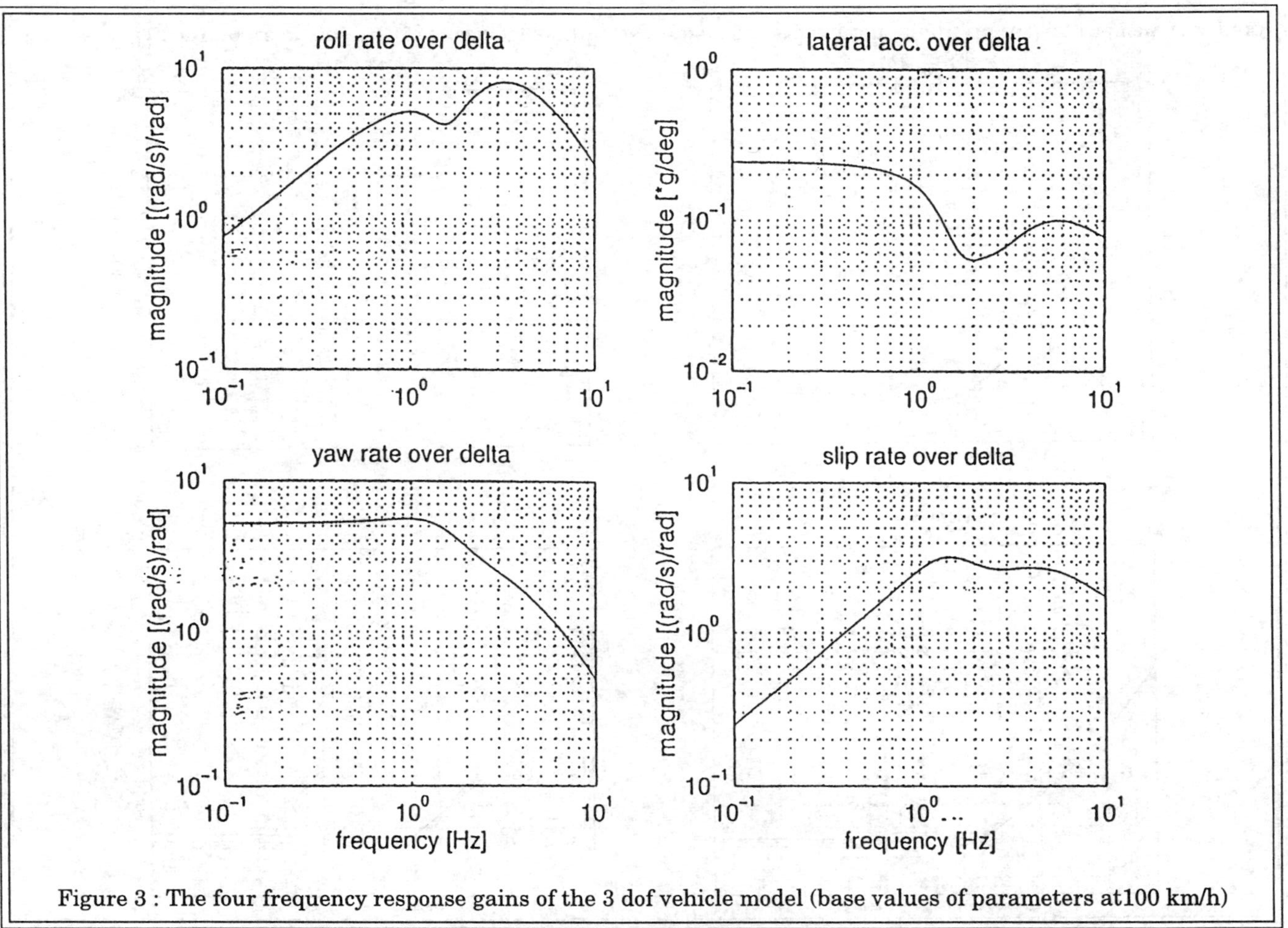

Figure 3 : The four frequency response gains of the 3 dof vehicle model (base values of parameters at100 km/h)

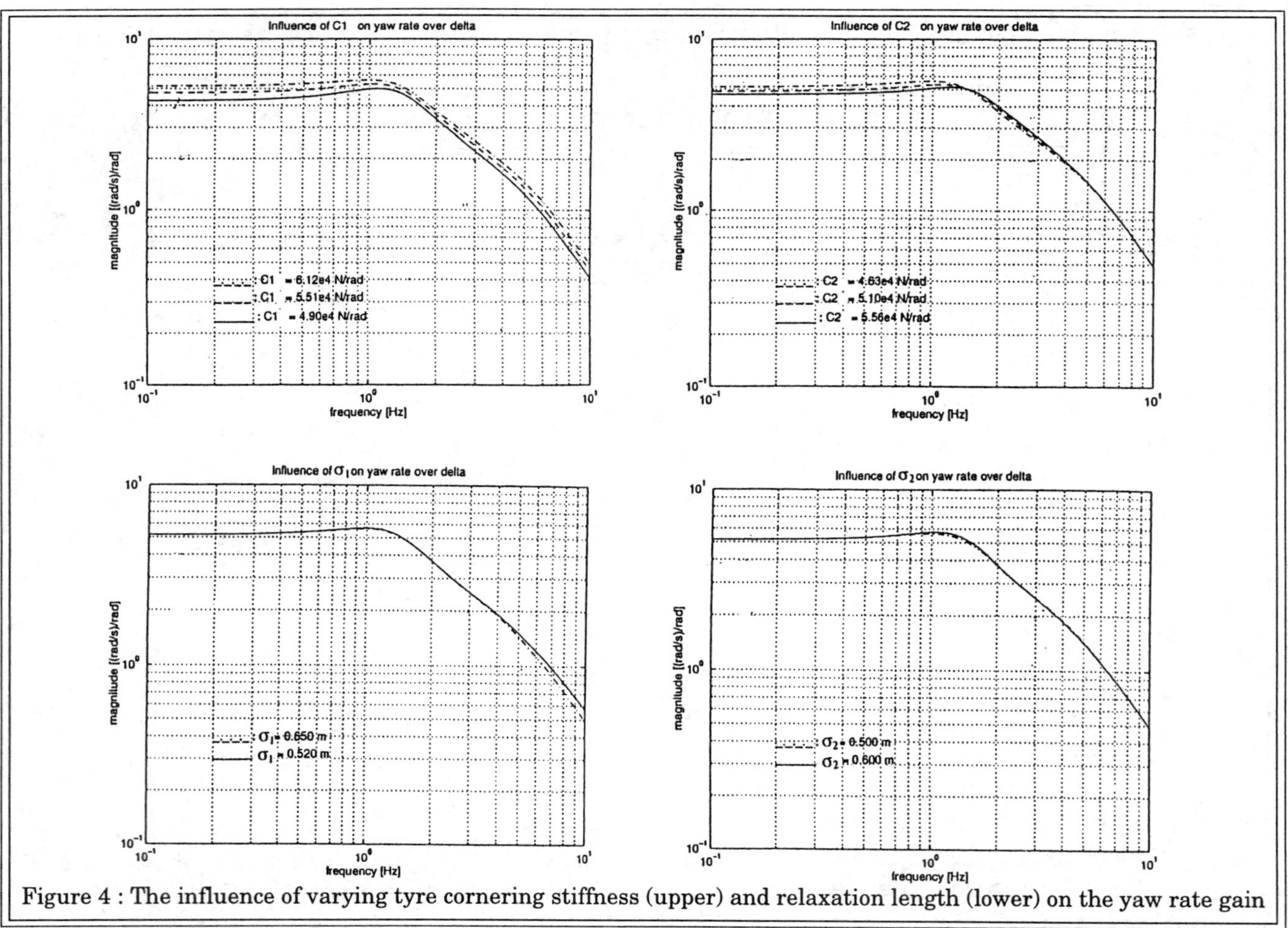

Figure 4 : The influence of varying tyre cornering stiffness (upper) and relaxation length (lower) on the yaw rate gain

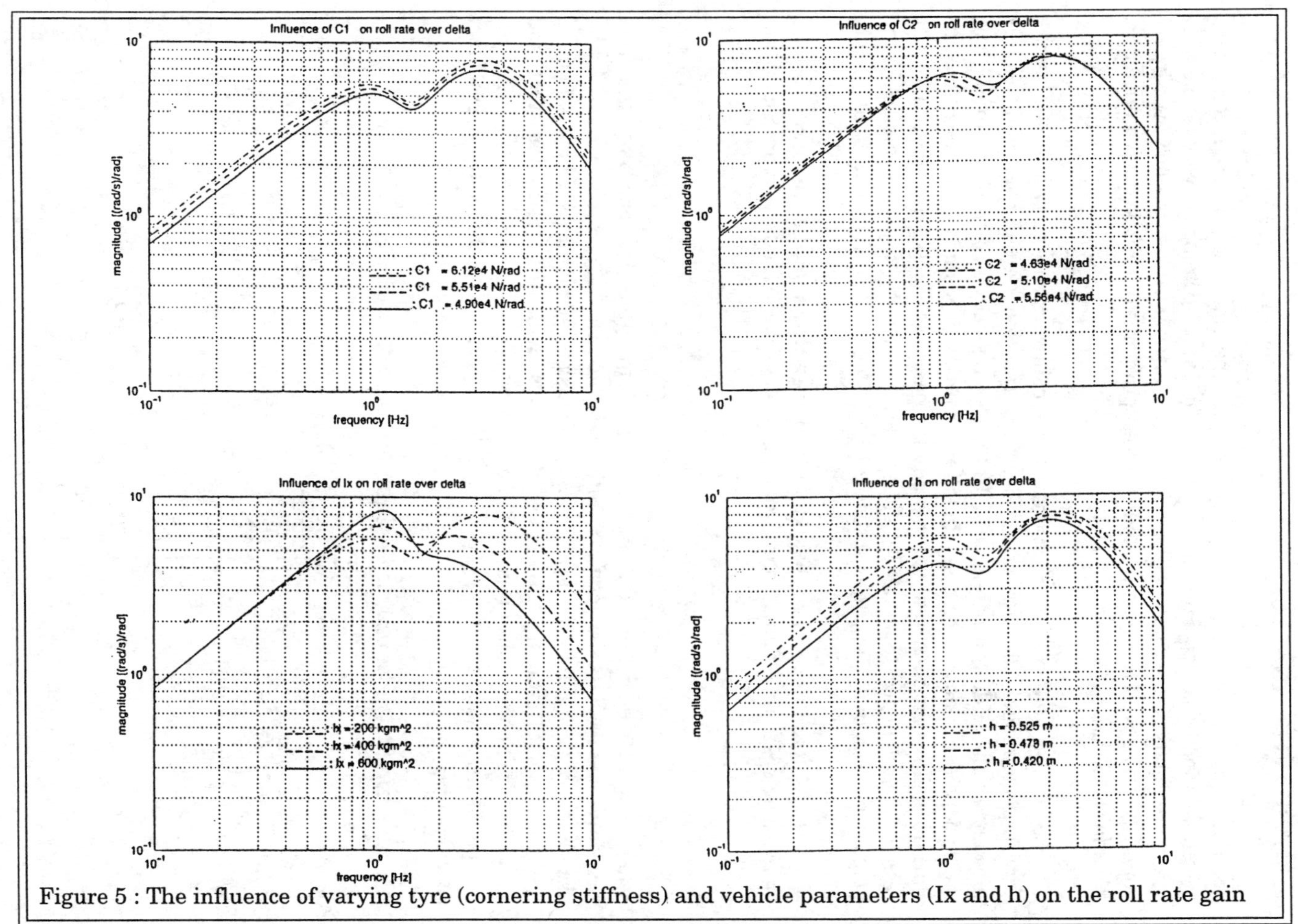

Figure 5 : The influence of varying tyre (cornering stiffness) and vehicle parameters (Ix and h) on the roll rate gain

4. SENSITIVITY ANALYSIS

As noted by Frank [12], sensitivity analysis provides design engineers with systematic methods for investigating the effects of parameter variations. The sensitivity analysis may be put to use in several different ways as illustrated by its application by several authors to study various problems of vehicle design related to dynamics [13-16].

This section presents results of a parametric sensitivity analysis of a 3-DOF linear yaw in-plane model. The first order sensitivity functions are derived with respect to several vehicle design parameters. Both the frequency response sensitivity and the real time response sensitivity functions have been studied. The sensitivity in time domain is particularly suited to study the parameter sensitivity of the transient response of vehicles to a rapid change in the steering input. The first order percentage sensitivity functions discussed by Nalecz [13 b] form the basis of this analysis.

The general definition of the sensitivity functions is determined as follows:

In the state-space time domain the dynamics of the vehicle model is represented by:

$$\dot{x} = f(x,p,t), \qquad x^{(0)} = x(t=0)$$

where $x = (x_1, x_2, x_3, ...x_n)^T$ is the state vector, (the dot represents the time derivative and the x^0 is the vector of initial values of x),

the function vector $f = (f_1, f_2, f_3, ...f_n)^T$ consists of elements which could be generally some arbitrary non-linear functions with the restriction that the derivatives are continuous in the region of interest.,

the parameter vector $p = (p_1, p_2, p_3, ...p_m)^T$ is a vector with the system parameters as elements.

The standard first order parameter sensitivity matrix S is defined by

$$S = \frac{\partial x}{\partial p} = \begin{bmatrix} \dfrac{\partial x_{(1)}}{\partial p_{(1)}} & \dfrac{\partial x_{(1)}}{\partial p_{(2)}} & \cdots & \dfrac{\partial x_{(1)}}{\partial p_{(m)}} \\[2mm] \dfrac{\partial x_{(2)}}{\partial p_{(1)}} & \dfrac{\partial x_{(2)}}{\partial p_{(2)}} & \cdots & \dfrac{\partial x_{(2)}}{\partial p_{(m)}} \\[2mm] \vdots & \vdots & \ddots & \vdots \\[2mm] \dfrac{\partial x_{(n)}}{\partial p_{(1)}} & \dfrac{\partial x_{(n)}}{\partial p_{(2)}} & \cdots & \dfrac{\partial x_{(n)}}{\partial p_{(m)}} \end{bmatrix}$$

The elements $S_{j,k}$ of this matrix are the standard first order sensitivity functions (of the variable x_k with respect to parameter p_j).
Taking the partial derivative of S with respect to the parameter vector p:

$$\dot{S} = \frac{\partial f}{\partial x} \cdot \frac{\partial x}{\partial p} + \frac{\partial f}{\partial p} = \frac{\partial f}{\partial x} S + \frac{\partial f}{\partial p}$$

In the present case of a 3 dof model of the vehicle the state vector x, and the steering control input u are

$$\overline{x}^T = \begin{vmatrix} \beta & r & p & \varphi & F_{y1} & F_{y2} \end{vmatrix}; \qquad \overline{u} = \delta$$

and the linearised equations of motion in the state space are

$$\dot{\overline{x}} = A\overline{x} + B\overline{u}$$

where the system matrix A of the 3 dof model is specified in the appendix.

The sensitivity differential becomes:

$$\dot{S} = A^{(0)} S + \left.\frac{\partial A}{\partial p}\right|_{p=p_0} x^{(0)} + \left.\frac{\partial B}{\partial p}\right|_{p=p_0} u \qquad S^{(0)} = \frac{\partial x^{(0)}}{\partial p} S = 0$$

where $A^{(0)} = A(p_0)$ and $x^{(0)} = x(t, p_0)$.

The goal of the sensitivity analysis is to determine the effect of parametric changes on the state variables or on other secondary variables (a combination of state variables).

Time Domain Sensitivity Analysis of Vehicle Transient Response to Steering

The sensitivity functions S are calculated for the transient manoeuvre of the vehicle following a ramp-step steering input defined by:

$$\delta(t) = K\,t \ \text{ for } o < t < t_1 \qquad \text{and} \qquad \delta(t) = K t_1 \ \text{ for } t_2 > t > t_1 .$$

The analysis is performed for a ramp-step steering input at a forward speed of 100 km/h in order to investigate the effects of small parameter variations on the transient response of yaw, side-slip and roll motion.

For numerical simulations the ramp-step steer input applied to the front road wheel had a step height of magnitude 1^0 and the total duration of input of 5 seconds was chosen so that the vehicle response approached quasi steady- state conditions.

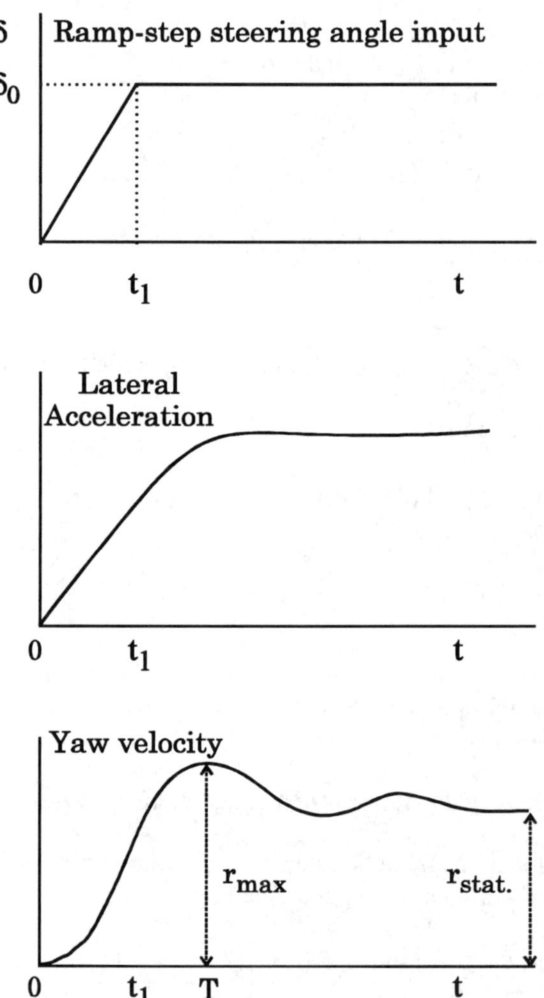

Figure 6: The ramp-step steering test-input and the lateral and yaw response.

Percentage Sensitivity Functions:

Instead of calculating the standard first-order sensitivity function S, it is more useful for engineering usage to obtain expressions for the percentage sensitivity function. In particular the percentage sensitivity facilitates comparison of changes in a system variable due to a user specified percentage change in the system parameters. The percentage sensitivity makes it easy to interpret the relative influence of different parameters on a particular response variable in identical units. The first order percentage sensitivity %S is defined by:

$$S^{\%} = \frac{\partial x}{\partial p}\, \delta p \quad \Rightarrow \quad S^{\%}{}_{j,k} = \frac{\xi\, p_j\, S_{j,k}}{x_k}$$

where ξ is the percentage change of the parameter p_j., being varied, the element $S_{j,k}$ is the first order standard sensitivity function which has been defined already and x_k is the variable influenced. This percentage function is convenient for comparing the effect of various parameters of the system on x_k.
The three response variables being investigated in this work are :

1) the side-slip angle of the body β
2) the yaw angular velocity r, and,
3) the roll angle φ

The percentage sensitivity has been calculated for a total number of 21 parameters. The majority of the 21 parameters are the main parameters of the vehicle model (Figure 2) used in the analysis described above The few remaining parameters have been introduced later in order to carry out a more detailed design analysis using a slightly more elaborate version of the 3 dof vehicle model in figure .
For convenience the 21 parameters are grouped into four categories.

Vehicle Parameters:
m: the total mass of the vehicle.
a: the distance along the x-axis between the front axle and the cg.
b: the distance along the x-axis between the rear axle and the cg.
h: the height of the cg above the road.
I_x : the moment of inertia about the X axis (roll).
I_z : the moment of inertia about the Z axis (yaw).

Suspension Kinematics Parameters:
ε_1 ,ε_2 : the front, rear roll steer coupling coefficients.
τ_1 ,τ_2 : the front and rear roll camber coupling coefficients.
F_{t1} , F_{t2} : the front and rear train local yaw flexibility's.

Vehicle Roll Parameters:
h_1 and h_2 : Vertical distance (parallel to the z axis) from the cg to the front and rear roll centres.
k the total roll damping rate.
Cr_1 and Cr_2 : the front and roll stiffness (total roll stiffness $c = Cr_1 + Cr_2$)

Tyre Parameters:
C_1 and C_2: the cornering stiffness of the front and rear tires.
σ_1 and σ_2 : the relaxation lengths of the front and rear tires.

In figures 7 - 9 results are presented for the first order percentage sensitivity functions of the body side-slip angle, yaw rate and the roll angle of the vehicle for the four categories of parameters. The absolute values of the motion variables for the baseline vehicle are shown by the dotted lines in the figures.

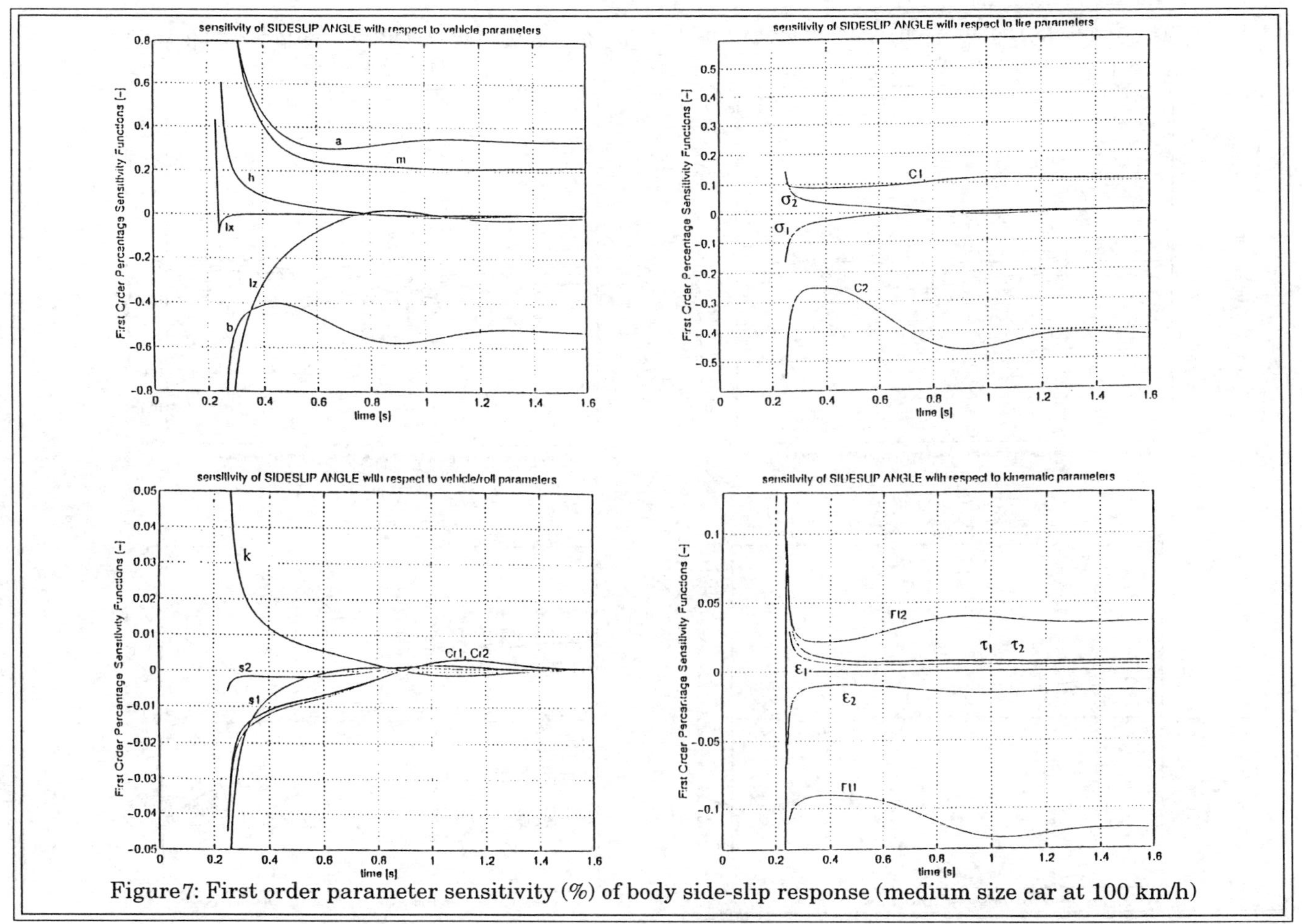

Figure 7: First order parameter sensitivity (%) of body side-slip response (medium size car at 100 km/h)

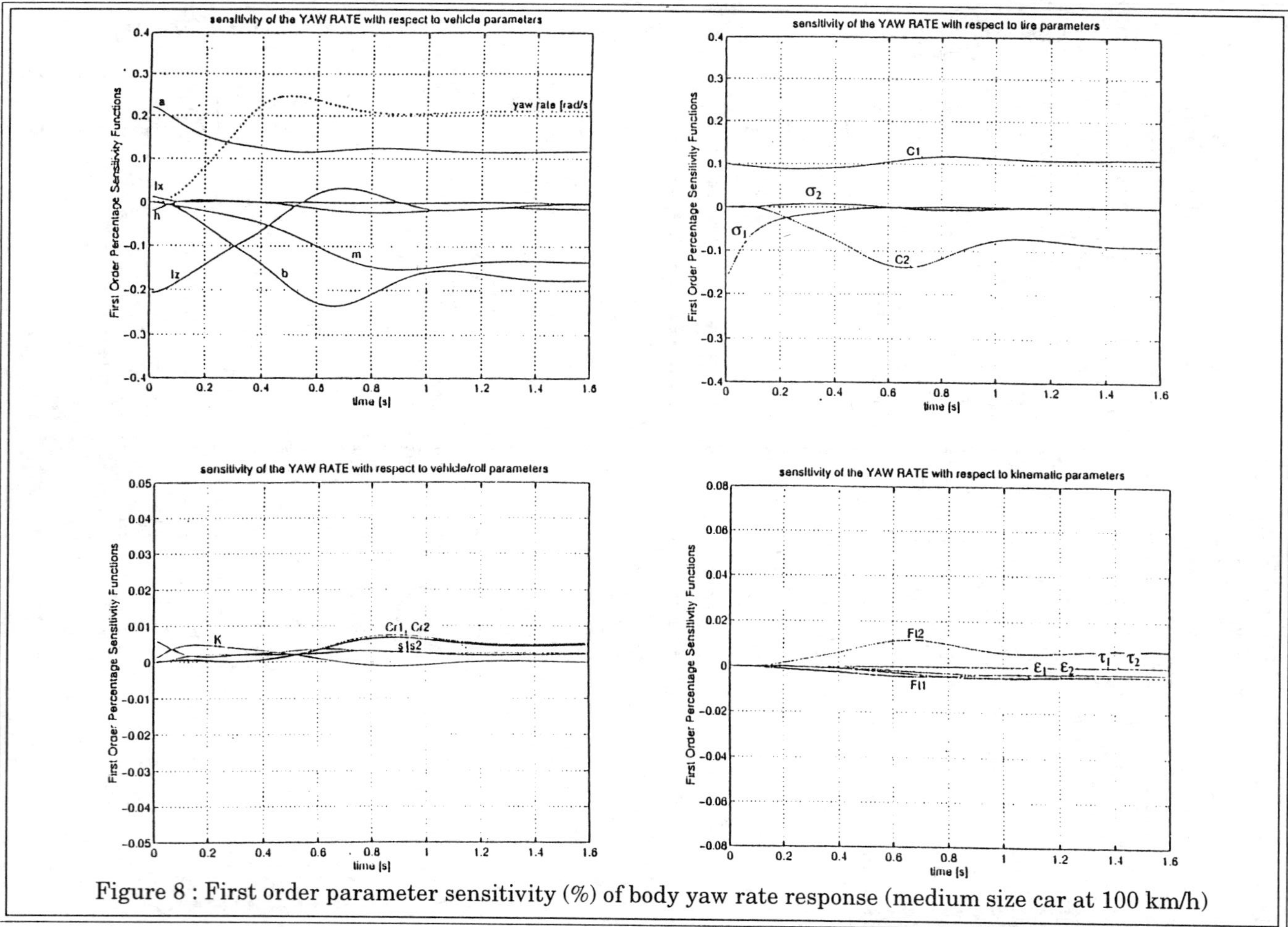

Figure 8 : First order parameter sensitivity (%) of body yaw rate response (medium size car at 100 km/h)

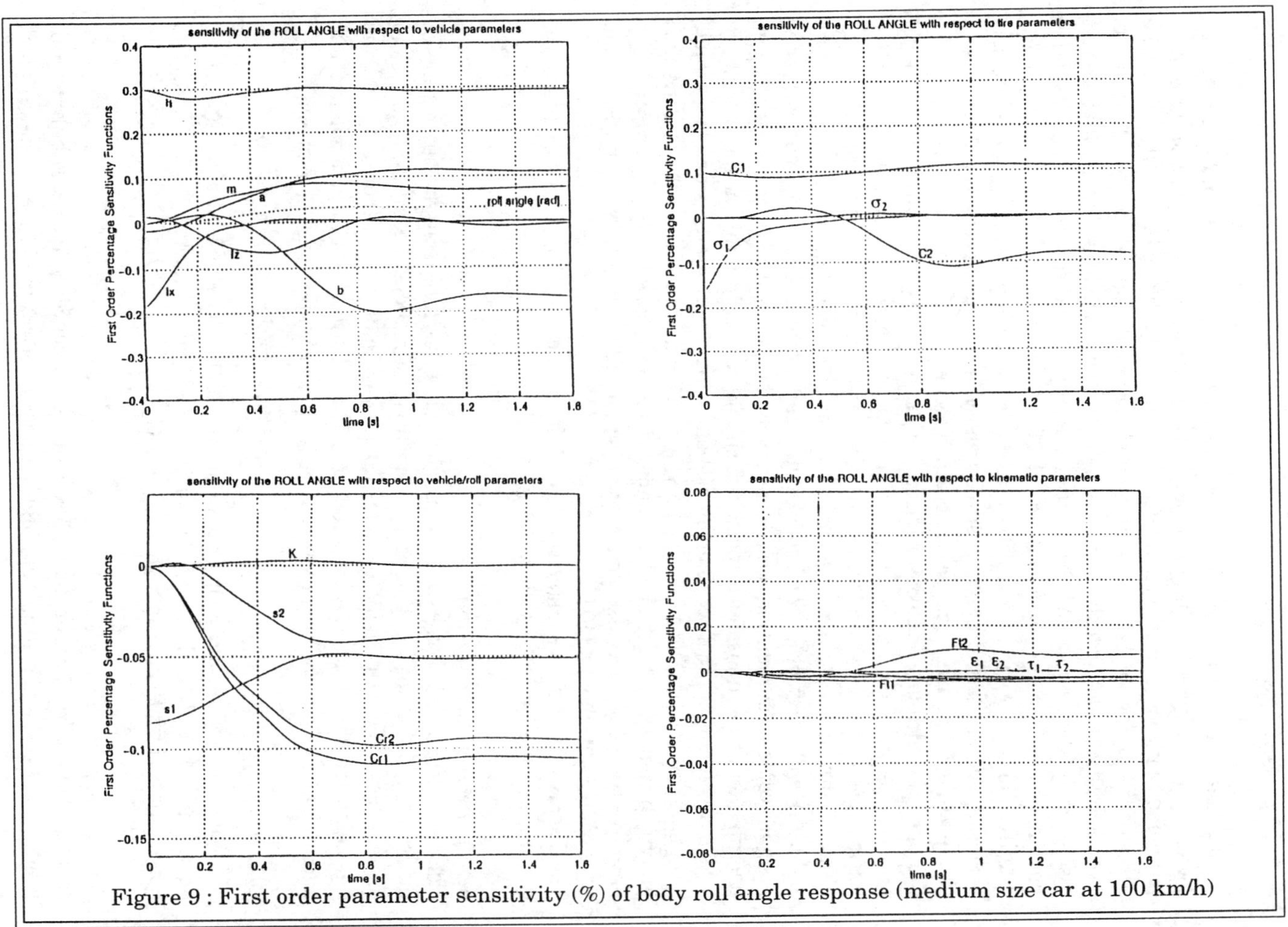

Figure 9 : First order parameter sensitivity (%) of body roll angle response (medium size car at 100 km/h)

5. CONCLUSIONS

In the light of the (demanding) the feed-forward and feedback control activities of the driver in transient handling manoeuvres and the information processing tasks it is argued that the subjective human judgement of the handling quality of vehicle depends mainly on the basic vehicle motion namely the lateral (body side slip), the yaw and the roll. Transient handling in various environmental situations is discussed in the context of the control strategy of the driver and the dynamic interaction between the driver and the vehicle.

The dynamics of a simple 3 dof bicycle model of a medium size passenger car is analysed. As an illustration, a sensitivity analysis the basic response of a medium size passenger car has been presented in frequency and time domains. Using the example of a medium size passenger car the transient response of the 3 dof model to a ramp-step steering input is calculated and the time domain percentage sensitivity functions are determined. The percentage sensitivity functions are plotted as functions of time for three key variables of vehicle motion (side slip, yaw and roll) with respect to 21 model parameters subdivided into four categories (overall vehicle, suspension kinematics, vehicle roll and tyre parameters). The presentation of the transient response sensitivity results in terms of the percentage sensitivity functions in time domain is both simple and useful from the vehicle designer's viewpoint. The side-slip and yaw rate are generally sensitive to variations in tyre parameters. A detailed account of the influence of tyre parameters on objective and subjective assessment of vehicle handling is discussed in the present volume by Pauwelussen [17].

The results of sensitivity analysis of the 3 dof model of a medium size passenger car may be summarised as follows:

Sensitivity of the side slip angle β:
The side slip angle becomes zero approximately 0.2 s following the application of the steering input.so the percentage sensitivity functions become singular and meaningless. The sensitivity of side-slip to yaw moment of inertia I_z and the relaxation lengths σ_1 and σ_2 is strong but it is of a highly transient nature. The ranking order of parameters in terms of the influence on β is: b, C_2 , a, m and C_1 .

Sensitivity of the yaw rate r:
The parameters a, σ_1 and I_z have a strong but highly transient influence (t<0.1 s) on r. Parameters I_z and and σ_1 have practically no influence for t>0.7 s. The ranking order of influence is b, m, a, C_1 and C_2.

Sensitivity of the roll angle φ:
As expected the height h of the cg has a strong influence on the sensitivity to roll. While I_x and σ_1 have a strong but highly transient effect the influence on response

becomes insignificant for $t > 0.4$ s. The influence of I_z is also felt in this highly transient due to the interaction between roll and yaw motion phase (although of a slightly longer duration than that due to I_x). The ranking order in this case: h, b, C_1, C_2, Ix, σ_1.

Clearly, the paper presents only a beginning of an approach towards objective assessment of vehicle handling in transient manoeuvres. Several important aspects of the transient response and sensitivity such as the response to driving and braking force inputs and to cross winds remain to be investigated.

APPENDIX

In the state space format the vectors of state and control variables and matrices are:

$$\bar{x}^T = \begin{vmatrix} \beta & r & p & \varphi & F_{y1} & F_{y2} \end{vmatrix}$$

$$\bar{u} = \delta \tag{3.6}$$

$$\bar{y}^T = \begin{vmatrix} \beta & r & p & \varphi \end{vmatrix}$$

$$A = \begin{vmatrix} a_{11} & a_{12} & a_{13} & a_{14} & a_{15} & a_{16} \\ a_{21} & a_{22} & a_{23} & a_{24} & a_{25} & a_{26} \\ a_{31} & a_{32} & a_{33} & a_{34} & a_{35} & a_{36} \\ a_{41} & a_{42} & a_{43} & a_{44} & a_{45} & a_{46} \\ a_{51} & a_{52} & a_{53} & a_{54} & a_{55} & a_{56} \\ a_{61} & a_{62} & a_{63} & a_{64} & a_{65} & a_{66} \end{vmatrix}$$

whose elements read

$$a_{11} = 0, a_{12} = -1, a_{13} = 0, a_{14} = 0, a_{15} = \frac{1}{mV}, a_{16} = \frac{1}{mV}$$

$$a_{21} = 0, a_{22} = 0, a_{23} = \frac{-kI_{xz}}{I_xI_z - I_{xz}^2}, a_{24} = \frac{-cI_{xz}}{I_xI_z - I_{xz}^2}, a_{25} = \frac{h_1I_{xz} + aI_x}{I_xI_z - I_{xz}^2}, a_{26} = \frac{h_2I_{xz} - bI_x}{I_xI_z - I_{xz}^2}$$

$$a_{31} = 0, a_{32} = 0, a_{33} = \frac{-kI_z}{I_xI_z - I_{xz}^2}, a_{34} = \frac{-cI_z}{I_xI_z - I_{xz}^2}, a_{35} = \frac{h_1I_z + aI_{xz}}{I_xI_z - I_{xz}^2}, a_{36} = \frac{h_2I_z - bI_{xz}}{I_xI_z - I_{xz}^2}$$

$$a_{41} = 0, a_{42} = 0, a_{43} = 1, a_{44} = 0, a_{45} = 0, a_{46} = 0$$

$$a_{51} = -\frac{C_1 V}{\sigma_1},\ a_{52} = -\frac{aC_1}{\sigma_1},\ a_{53} = -\frac{h_1 C_1}{\sigma_1},\ a_{54} = \frac{(\varepsilon_1 C_1 + \tau_1 C_{\gamma 1})V}{\sigma_1},\ a_{55} = -\frac{V}{\sigma_1},\ a_{56} = 0$$

$$a_{61} = -\frac{C_2 V}{\sigma_2},\ a_{62} = \frac{bC_2}{\sigma_2},\ a_{63} = -\frac{h_2 C_2}{\sigma_2},\ a_{64} = \frac{(\varepsilon_2 C_2 + \tau_2 C_{\gamma 2})V}{\sigma_2},\ a_{65} = 0,\ a_{66} = -\frac{V}{\sigma_2}$$

The input matrix

$$B = \begin{bmatrix} b_1 & b_2 & b_3 & b_4 & b_5 & b_6 \end{bmatrix}$$

where $b_1 = 0, b_2 = 0, b_3 = 0, b_4 = 0, b_5 = \dfrac{C_1 V}{\sigma_1}, b_6 = 0$

$$C = \begin{vmatrix} 1 & 0 & 0 & 0 & 0 & 0 \\ 0 & 1 & 0 & 0 & 0 & 0 \\ 0 & 0 & 1 & 0 & 0 & 0 \\ 0 & 0 & 0 & 1 & 0 & 0 \end{vmatrix} \qquad D = \begin{vmatrix} 0 \\ 0 \\ 0 \\ 0 \end{vmatrix}$$

REFERENCES

[1] Apetauer, M and Opicka, F., "Assessment of the driver's effort in typical manoeuvres for different vehicle configurations and managements", Proc. of the 12 th IAVSD symposium on the dynamics of vehicles on roads and on rails, Lyon (France), ed. G. Sauvage, Supplement to Vehicle System Dynamics Vol. 20, (1991), pp. 42-56.

[2] Sharp, R.S., " Vehicle dynamics and the judgement of quality", in the present volume.

[3] Kageyama, I and Pacejka, H.B., "On a new driver model with fuzzy control", Proc. IAVSD symposium on the dynamics of vehicles on roads and on rails, Lyon (France), ed. G. Sauvage, Supplement to Vehicle System Dynamics Vol. 20,(1991), pp. 314-324.

[4] Gu Xi and Yu Qun, "Driver-vehicle-environment closed loop simulation of handling and stability using fuzzy conrol theory ", Proc. of the 13th IAVSD symposium on the dynamics of vehicles on roads and on rails, Chengdu (P.R.China), ed. Z. Shen, Supplement to Vehicle System Dynamics Vol. 23 (1993), pp. 172-181.

[5] Yoshimoto, K., "Course tracking algorithm using visual information", Vehicle System Dynamics, 28, No. 6, Dec. (1997), pp 385-398.

[6] Mitschke, M., "Dynamik der Kraftfahrzeug", Band C: Fahrverhalten, Springer-Verlag, (1990).

[7] Loos, H. and Dödlbacher, G., "A mathematical "prototype" of the vehicle to describe vehicle handling behaviour", Proc. of 9th IAVSD symposium on the dynamics of vehicles on roads and on rails, Linchöping (Sweden), ed. O. Nordström, Supplement to Vehicle System Dynamics Vol. 15, (1985), pp. 320-341.

[8] Furukawa, Y., Yuhara, N., Sano, S., Takeda, H. and Matsushita, Y., "Ä review of four-wheel steering studies from the viewpoint of vehicle dynamics and control", Vehicle System Dynamics, 18, (1989), pp. 151-186.

[9] Furukawa, Y. and Abe, M., "Advanced chassis control systems for vehicle handling and active safety", Vehicle System Dynamics, Vol. 28, (1997), pp. 59-86.

[10] Nakagawa, J., Tanaka, M and Yoshimoto K, "Modelling of a driver's behaviour considering roll motion", JSAE Review (Elsevier), 15, (1994), pp. 35-43.

[11] Pasterkamp, W.B. and Pacejka H.B., "The tyre as a sensor to estimate friction", Vehicle System Dynamics, Vol. 27, No. 5-6, June (1995), pp 725-758

[12] Frank, P.M., Introduction to system sensitivity theory", Academic Press, (1978).

[13 a] Nalecz, A.G. "Sensitivity analysis of vehicle design attributes infrequency domain", Vehicle System Dynamics, Vol. 17, No. 3, (1988), pp. 141-163

[13 b] Nalecz A.G. "Application of sensitivity methods to analysis and synthesis of vehicle dynamic systems", Vehicle System Dynamics, Vol.18, No. 1-3, (1989), pp.1-44.

[14] Sharp, R S.and Brooks, P.C., "Sensitivities of frequency response functions of linear dynamic systems to variations in design parameters"' J. Sound and Vibration, 26, (1988), pp. 167-172.

[15] Horton, D.N.L., and Crolla, D.A., "Application of linear sensitivity methods to vehicle dynamics problems", Proc. IAVSD symposium on the dynamics of vehicles on roads and on rails, Lyon (France), ed. G. Sauvage, Supplement to Vehicle System Dynamics Vol. 20, (1991), pp. 269-283.

[16] Palkovic, L and El-Gindy, M., "Design of an active unilateral brake control system for five-axle tractor semi-trailer based on sensitivity analysis", Vehicle System Dynamics, 24, (1995), pp 725-758

[17] Pauwelussen, J., "Effect of tyre handling characteristics on driver judgement of vehicle directional stability" in the present volume.

Session:

Design, Sensitivity Analysis and Applications

Effect of Tyre Handling Characteristics on Driver Judgement of Vehicle Directional Stability

Joop P. Pauwelussen

There is no doubt that tyres have a strong impact on vehicle behaviour and on the driver assessment of vehicle performance. This relates to handling, perceived safety and controllability, the amount of effort required to react, course following and straight line stability, etc.
Several of these aspects are known to correlate to some extent with objective indicators such as gains, response times and alike, as obtained from open loop reference tests. But there is more, particularly in relation to the interface between steering system and the driver control and perceived feed-back, where these phenomena are still not well understood. In fact, this was one of the motivations for the seminar "Understanding Human Monitoring and Assessment".

In the paper, several studies from the past are discussed focusing on the influence of tyre design parameters on the driver assessment, where both open-loop and closed-loop results are considered. This results in an overview of the discriminating physical tyre parameters examined, the experimental approaches applied, and the outputparameters (subjective and objective identifiers) describing the vehicle behaviour.

These studies start with variation in quantities such as tyre pressure, compound, age (effect of tyre wear), geometry whereas vehicle handling simulation studies deal with performance characteristics in terms of cornering stiffness, pneumatic trail, etc. exploiting for example the scaling factors in the Delft-Tyre Magic Formula model. Mathematical studies are suited for interpretation of vehicle handling performance in terms of such tyre characteristics (e.g. Magic Formula model data). This means that, in order to use these studies for further investigating the impact of tyre characteristics on driver assessment, relationships between tyre design parameters and performance characteristics are required.

Using a simple simulation model, derived from and validated by realistic vehicle characteristic data from the TNO Vehicle Dynamic Database, the effect of some of these tyre performance characteristics has been examined based on the vehicle lateral frequency response and transient response behaviour while turning into a curve (J-turn). The results of these simulation studies are discussed, also referring to the subjective and objective correlation results as resulting from the literature survey. It is recognised that the level of complexity of the simulation model is not appropriate to study the sensitivity of the driver opinion on tyre performance in all its detail. Some conclusions will be drawn within this respect, and ideas about a further follow-up will be presented.

1. INTRODUCTION

In order to understand the behaviour of a driver-vehicle system under normal or emergency conditions, the role of the tyre is of outmost importance. Tyres keep the vehicle on the road under extreme manoeuvring by the driver in response of unexpected situations, they assist the driver in predicting the performance of his vehicle under such conditions, they

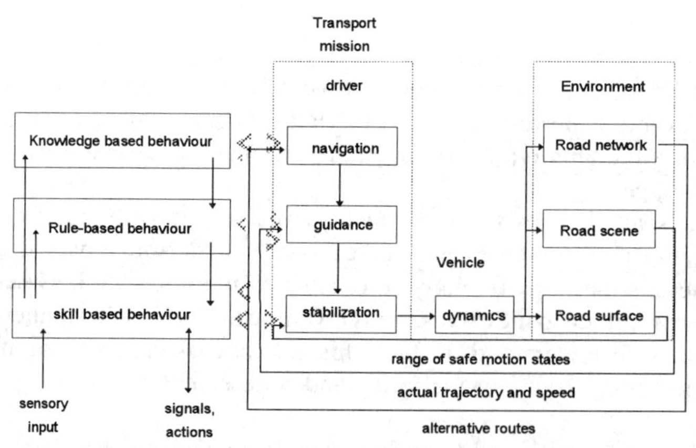

Figure 1.: Human behaviour and driving tasks [3]

confirm him that he is still in control, they inform him about deviations from an intended path through the steering system, that means that they serve to preview and warn for danger ahead, etc. This means that tyres work out on the driver perception and response at different levels. These levels can be considered with reference to the categories of human behaviour and driving task hierarchy as distinguished by Donges [3] and depicted in fig. 1. At the left of this figure, the classic hierarchy in behavioural categories is shown with distinction between **knowledge based behaviour** corresponding to the response to unfamiliar situations, **rule-based behaviour** corresponding to associative response based on selection of the most appropriate alternative according to earlier subjective experience, and **skill-based behaviour** which can be regarded as an automatic, unconscious reflex. Comparing this classification to the different driving task levels as shown in figure 1, tyres are mainly of relevance at the levels indicated as **guidance** and **stabilisation**. The dynamic status of the vehicle involves changes in the input data for the driver, a major part of which is effected by the tyres (steering feel, vibrations, noise, lateral motions, etc.). The driver responds partly at guidance level (such as corresponding to open loop control) and partly at stabilisation level (such as corresponding to closed loop control). The distinction between those two levels depends on the driver and his experience with similar traffic situations. At the lowest level, information is obtained through the dynamics of the vehicle, yielding a perceived friction level, road-wheel contact, road unevenness, resulting cornering and braking resistance on basis of which the driver has to decide, consciously or unconsciously, about safe versus unsafe conditions and the necessary measures to overcome the endangered circumstances. Anticipation of forthcoming situations will improve the driver's response, and his ability to avoid accidents.

Another schematic overview of the driver's actions to emergency situations has been given by Braun and Ihme and reported by Käppler and Godthelp in [6], see fig. 2. The three "partners" in any arbitrary traffic situation indicated in the right part of figure 1, i.e. driver, vehicle and environment, are shown in figure 2 as contributors to an experienced level of risk. Such "latent risks" could be effected by poor driving behaviour (like excessive speed), a vehicle deficiency (e.g. low tyre pressure) or changes in the environment (slippery road, poor visibility, dense traffic,...). Reduced safety margins under typical adverse road- and weather conditions have been studied within the DRIVE project ROSES (ROad Safety Enhancement Systems), where not only single causes but also combinations of different hazards have been considered [13]. A sudden event may yield a sharp increase in risk level and, as a consequence, a reduced stabilising tolerance, that is a return to the original risk level. After some reaction time the driver may intervene correctly, he may intervene incorrectly (braking on an icy surface) or he may not respond or respond too late if the accident level has already been reached.

Again, it is clear that appropriate information that is based, to a large extent, on tyre performance would help the driver to anticipate risky situations (i.e. reduce the reaction time), whereas the driver-vehicle system performance is crucial to overcome emergency situations.

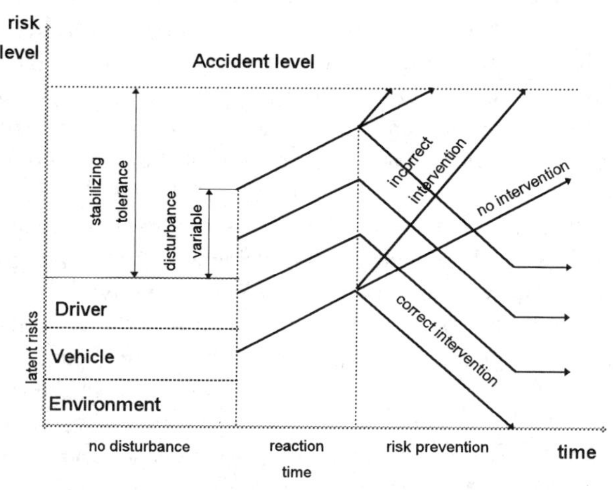

Figure 2.: Driver response to potentially dangerous situations [6]

The approaches as outlined above support the conclusions that the tyre-road interface characteristics affect vehicle handling qualities and constitute, through these, a critical factor in the risk reduction potential at critical situations. They contribute to the driver input and the driver's ability to take appropriate corrective measure to avoid potential crash conditions. As an example one may think of the steeringwheel torque feedback, which depends on the non-linear characteristics of tyres and suspension, and which may contribute to the subjective rating of the control behaviour. This example illustrates the interaction of tyre response with other vehicle subsystems, making it more difficult to obtain a clear understanding of the impact of tyre characteristics on driver judgement and control.

There is yet another more economic reason to look more closely into the driver assessment of tyre characteristics. In the automotive industry there is a strong desire for further improvement of the safety and handling qualities of vehicles, both under normal and extreme operational conditions. As a consequence of this development, vehicle manufacturers presently put increasing demands on the various parts of a vehicle (such as suspension and tyres) in order to guarantee the optimal vehicle handling and safety qualities as envisaged in the vehicle design. Since most of the verification of vehicle performance qualities is based on human judgement, a better understanding of the driver monitoring and assessment process will contribute to an improved vehicle-driver response and a more efficient and effective design process. In particular, this is true when the additional benefits of introducing advanced control concepts as part of new designs are considered, with the objective to improve or maintain the safety of the vehicle under a wide range of driving conditions. One may think of developments related to yaw moment control (VDC, EPS,..) and other slip-control systems to understand that the tyre road interface plays a dominant role here.

The success of critical automotive component design (either related to the tyre/suspension part, or to advanced vehicle control systems) is determined to a large extent by the integrated behaviour of the component-vehicle-driver system. When analysing these developments from an engineering, marketing or business point of view, considering the fact that basically, evaluations are subjective, business risks are implied for a manufacturer when investing in these developments. This situation may be relieved by expanding the knowledge about the human judgement of critical vehicle qualities. Research in the area of human assessment of vehicle performance may lead to a further understanding of the criteria of assessment of an experienced or inexperienced driver in his judgement of vehicle properties.

These considerations lead to the following objectives for this paper:

- to contribute in understanding of the impact of tyre characteristics on driver judgement
- to explore the state of the art in the subjective assessment of tyre performance
- to explore potentially appropriate methodologies that could be successfully exploited for further research in this field

The paper is organised as follows. In section 2, some previous studies are outlined, where distinction is made between the input tyre characteristics and the output vehicle performance parameters with emphasis on the relationship between subjective and objective assessment. Next, in section 3, the variation of tyre characteristics will be treated in terms of the Magic Formula tyre model, with reference to the selected scaling factors which were specially introduced for this purpose. In section 4, simulation studies are reported where the sensitivity of vehicle performance with respect to certain tyre characteristics is treated for a simple vehicle simulation model, both in the frequency domain and the time domain (restricted to the step-steer response). Results are discussed in section 5, with some ideas for further investigations. Finally, conclusions are drawn up in section 6.

2. HUMAN MONITORING AND TYRE CHARACTERISTICS

Several papers have been published in the past on the impact of tyre characteristics on vehicle performance assessment and driver feedback information. These contributions have in common that the sensitivity of selected tyre parameters is investigated using objective or subjective assessment methods where, in some cases, correlations are identified between these open- and closed loop results. Hence, different tyre construction and performance parameters are distinguished (input tyre characteristics), different methodologies are explored related to certain vehicle handling tests, resulting into output parameters that are either connected to open-loop vehicle performance or subjective driver ratings.
In this order, the previous research results will be treated in the subsequent subsections, with a discussion on the impact of the various input tyre characteristics on vehicle performance in the final one. We start with a concise characterisation of each of the papers.

Roland et al [14] investigated the sensitivity of tyre design (construction, dimensions) and, through that, tyre performance parameters on the vehicle dynamic response. Both manoeuvring and braking were considered. Several testprocedures were discussed where some of them were considered not to be appropriate. Correlation between tyre design and vehicle performance appeared to be not clear in many cases, and it was concluded to emphasise directly, in future studies, on tyre performance parameters. Fairlie and Pottinger [4] considered tyres that varied with respect to hardness and hysteresis with the objective to recommend best practice subjective methodologies in order to discriminate between these tyres in terms of suggested handling rating characteristics. They identified the different sources of error in judgement and proposed certain "rules" to minimise these errors. Brindle [1,2] examined the effects of tyre type (radial vs. cross-ply) and tyre dimension (standard vs. low-profile) on vehicle steering and handling and the perception of the driver on these characteristics. Whereas radials were favoured with respect to feelings about safety, security, control in case of emergencies, cross-ply tyres were rated better concerning the "feel" from the road. Brindle concluded that "steering feel" should be further studied from a broader perspective accounting for steering work, driver feedback from the steering, linearity in response, etc. Käppler and Godthelp [6] examined the effect of tyre pressure variations (resulting in different cornering stiffness at front and rear) through both open and closed loop test procedures, as well as subjective rating procedures to verify earlier findings. This work links objective and subjective assessment procedures that should form the basis for further research on the understanding of the impact of tyre characteristics on driver-vehicle performance. Xia and Willis [17] focused on the tyre cornering stiffness and compared different evaluation methods to rank the tyres with respect to vehicle handling performance.

In addition to evaluation methods related to single performance parameters such as gain or response time, they considered four-parameter evaluation method attributed to Mimuro [9]. To some extent, this approach can be considered as an extension to the well known two-parameter evaluation method due to Weir and DiMarco [16].

We finally mention the project TIME, presently carried out under responsibility of TNO with involvement of a large number of tyre-manufacturers and vehicle manufacturers, with the objective to derive new types of tyre testing procedures that are more closely related to the behaviour of a tyre underneath a vehicle under realistic driving conditions. Different parameters are varied within TIME, including service temperature, which is of much relevance to the topic of this paper. Since TIME has not yet been finalised, results will be reported at later date.

2.1. INPUT TYRE CHARACTERISTICS

Tyre parameter	Additional remarks	References
Construction parameters:	hardness	[4]
Compound	hysteresis	[4]
	cross-ply vs. radial	[1, 14]
Ply-type	nylon, rayon, polyester	[14]
Carcass material	rayon, Fiberglas, steel	[14]
Belt material		
Dimensions:		
Size	-	[14]
Aspect ratio	standard vs. low profile tyre	[2, 14]
Service parameters:		
Inner pressure	incl. mixed conditions (front-	[6]
Temperature	rear)	TIME
Wet vs. dry conditions	-	[2, 14]
Performance parameters:	incl. mixed conditions (front-	[14,17]
Cornering stiffness	rear)	[17]
Aligning torque	-	[17]
Pneumatic trail	-	[14]
Peak lateral force coefficient	$(F_y / F_z)_{peak}$	[14]
Braking force coefficient	$(F_x / F_z)_{peak}$	
Ageing parameters:		
Wear after normal use	-	[6]
Wear-in	-	[14]

Table 1.: Input tyre characteristics

The various input tyre characteristics as discussed in literature are summarised in table 1. above.

Distinction is made between construction parameters, geometrical characteristics (dimensions), service parameters such as inner pressure, performance parameters, and ageing of the tyre referring to the effect of age and wear-in procedures on tyre performance characteristics. The tyre construction and geometry imply certain performance characteristics, where the understanding and exploitation of these relationships is one of the main challenges for a tyre manufacturer. With our nowadays tyre models, one is pretty much capable of examining vehicle response as a result of modified tyre performance characteristics (see also section 3). However, by the end of the day, a tyre manufacturer is faced with the task to manufacture a tyre satisfying such performance requirements. Some comments will be made on these issues in subsection 2.4.

Finally, we do not pretend to give a full account of the impact of all possible tyre parameters on vehicle-driver performance. For example, the effect of tread design, tyre width, relaxation length etc. are not treated here and open for further investigations. We refer also to the contribution of Savkoor, Happel and Horkay [15] in this same seminar for further information on some of the open spots in the present paper.

2.2. METHODOLOGIES

Methodologies on the assessment of vehicle performance can be structured as follows:

- **Subjective methodology strategies**
    - <u>Performance tests</u>
      Referring to a specific task as determining a maximum speed (lane change), minimum lateral deviations, steering motions (straight lane test), etc.,
    - <u>Rating scales</u> (based on a questionnaire) followed by data reduction (PCA: Principal Component Analysis, DFA: Discriminant Function Analysis).
    - <u>Open questions</u>, to be considered as additional to the previous two strategies.
- **Objective methodology strategies**
    - Reference Manoeuvres with instrumented vehicles

There doesn't seem to be a standard test procedure at hand, as illustrated from the tests as encountered in the literature and listed in tables 2 and 3, with some of the performance metrics indicated in the second column.

Subjective methodology strategies	Some performance metrics
Realistic driving conditions along mixed routes on public roads, including rural, suburban and motorway roads.	-
Closed loop straight lane driving test	lateral vehicle position, required steering inputs; both in amplitude and frequency.
Closed loop double lane change	

Table 2.: Subjective methodology strategies encountered in the literature

Objective methodology strategies	Some performance metrics
Random (or swept) steering input test, with frequency range between 0 and 2.5 Hz	phase lags, equivalent time lag, steady state gain; for yaw rate and lateral acceleration
Step steering input test	response times, overshoot values, TB-factor or "vehicle characteristic"
Pulse steer input(alternative to random steer test)	-
Trapezoidal steering input test	peak lateral acceleration, peak yaw and bodyslip angles, peak sideslip angular rate
Sinusoidal steering input test	similar to above
Steady state cornering test	understeer factor
Straight line braking	longitudinal average deceleration
Braking in a turn	deceleration, body slip angular rate and change in path curvature
Turning on a rough road	similar to above

Table 3.: Objective methodology strategies encountered in the literature

Subjective ratings consist of numerical values, provided by the testdrivers (subjects) for each characteristic from a predefined list, according to a scale of some magnitude. This could be a 5-point scale [1], a 10-point scale [4, 6].

One should be aware that not only the ratings itself are important but also the deviations among the ratings, allowing a distinction between **individual** assessments by the subjects and assessments with high level of **consistency**.

Usually, the set of original variables is reduced to a set of so-called Principal Components or factors which can be regarded as orthogonal (statistically independent) to each of the other components (PCA: Principal Component Analysis). Principal Components are weighted linear combinations of the original measured variables. A next step could then be to reduce this set to new linear combinations with maximum discrimination between two or more clusters (e.g.

related to tyres with high and low cornering stiffness). This second step is referred to as Discriminant Function Analysis (DFA). Some researchers skip the PCA-analysis and apply a direct reduction based on the criterium of maximum discrimination, followed by an interpretation towards more independent factors.

Carrying out such PCA-analysis on both open-loop test results and subjective ratings would allow for further correlation studies between the objective and subjective test procedures.

2.3. ASSESSMENT OF VEHICLE PERFORMANCE

There is a general understanding that for the evaluation of vehicle handling performance, the steady state gain between yaw rate and steering input, the response times after a step steer, and the equivalent time constant play an important role. Small values of phase lag in both yaw rate and lateral acceleration appear to correlate well with a positive driver judgement of vehicle controllability [17]. In addition, there is evidence that a small phase lag difference between the lateral acceleration and the yaw rate is appreciated by a driver as well. This indicator played an important role in the discussions on four-wheel steering, as well as the criterium of zero sideslip angle. In fact, it was found that, for example at a severe steering manoeuvre, a driver isn't able to distinguish properly between a nonzero sideslip angle and a delay in yawrate response. The highest correlation was found between subjective rating and the product of steady-state sideslip angle and yaw rate peak time as resulting from the step steer input test. This last combined parameter is usually referred to as the TB factor. Xia and Willis [17] refer to this parameter as the "vehicle characteristic".

According to the discussion in the preceding subsection, all of these parameters as derived from some of the tests in table 3, may be further combined into statistically independent factors that may predict certain aspects of driver judgement of vehicle performance.

The equivalent time constant, denoted as T_{eq}, is defined by the frequency at which the phase shift between steering angle and yaw rate amounts 45 °. This means that the equivalent time constant T_{eq} describes the required driver phase lag compensation and the vehicle's effective steering bandwidth. It was demonstrated by Weir and DiMarco [16] that the steady state yaw rate gain G_r should not be too high (to avoid nervous behaviour) and not be too low (to avoid excessive steering input). They determined optimal boundaries in the (T_{eq}, G_r) plane for expert and typical drivers, which were extended by Godthelp, Ruijs & v. Randwijk [5] for heavy vehicles. These boundaries, as indicated in figure 3, were derived based on a rating of 3.5 and higher on a 10-point scale.

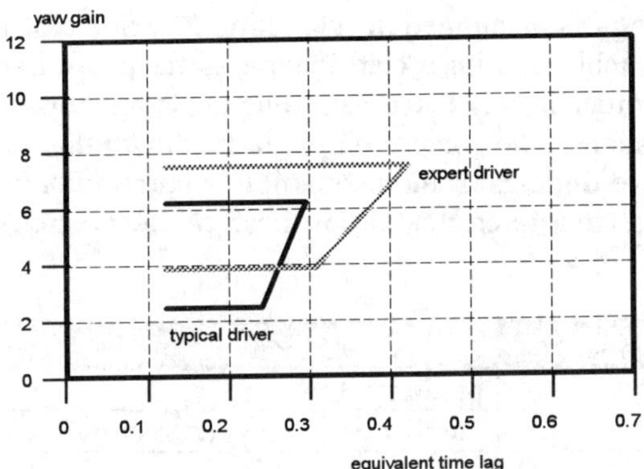

Figure 3.: Optimal handling boundaries [16]

Mimuro [9] extended the idea of multi-parameter evaluation to investigate vehicle handling qualities to a method including four parameters:

- G_r: steady state yaw rate gain
- ω_n: the yaw rate natural frequency
- ξ_r: the damping ratio for the yaw rate frequency response
- ϕ: phase lag of the lateral acceleration frequency response at 1 Hz

These four parameters together form a rhombus, as indicated in figure 4, where the area can be interpreted as a measure for linear vehicle handling potential. This approach has been applied by Xia et. al. [17] where the four parameters were obtained from fitting vehicle frequency response functions to the two degree of freedom "bicycle model", which appeared to work out very well. The most dominant factors turned out to be the natural frequency and the lateral acceleration phase lag, in discriminating between tyres with different cornering stiffness.

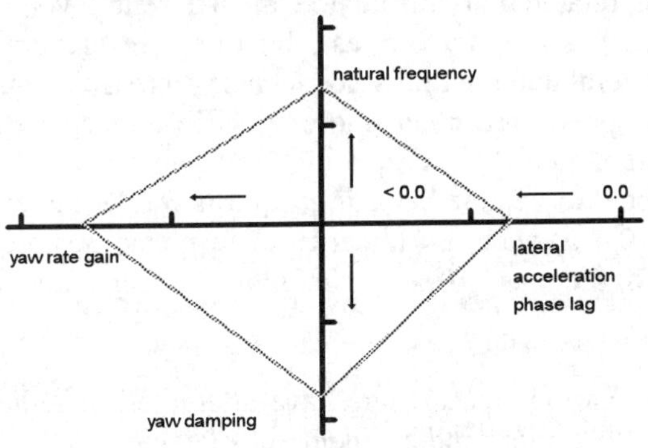

Figure 4.: Four parameter presentation [9]

Let us return to the subjective ratings as mentioned in subsection 2.2. Some of the characteristics have been listed in table 4, with a clarification as far as available from literature. There is no strict order in this list. Again, one observes a lack of standardisation in the type of questions. The conclusion might be drawn that only a thorough analysis of the subjective findings including possibly a correlation with objective results would allow for a clear interpretation of these characteristics, in retrospective.

Subjective characteristics (in random order)	
consequences of inattention	predictability
controllability	number of steering corrections
reaction accuracy	amount of steering angle
judgement about reaction speed	steering sensitivity
amount of steering force	steering reverse
reaction speed (to steering input)	handling in general
plowing (controllability vehicle front end)	swingout (controllability vehicle rear end)
tracking (maintain straight heading)	returnability (to original path)
perceived safety and security	perceived confidence (predictability)
sensitivity and lightness of steering	steering qualities in general
self-aligning strength of steering	vehicle stability
amount of effort while steering	linearity in response
amount of perceived feel through steering	amount of steering feel, thought ideal

Table 4.: Some subjective characteristics [1], [4], [6]

Clearly, the factors in table 4 are not independent. For example, "linearity in response" and "predictability" are related but formulated at different levels of perception. The same can be said about factors as "handling in general", "controllability" which are very general and qualitative concepts whereas "amount of effort of steering" or "reaction speed" are much more specific and closer to quantitative parameters as described earlier.
In addition, some factors are restricted to vehicle behaviour up to a moderate level of lateral acceleration (order 0.3 - 0.4 g) such as "linearity in response" whereas other factors are applicable up to the case of extreme manoeuvring such as "perceived safety and security".

Based on maximum discrimination, various researchers have attempted to reduce the set of subjective characteristics to a more independent set of factors, with or without a preceding orthogonalisation step. In this way, Brindle and Wilson [1] concluded that the perceived feel of safety and security (including control in emergency), stability and course following, the effort required to steer the vehicle and the "feel" through the steering system were most appropriate to predict the ranking between different tyre types. Fairlie and Pottinger [4] arrived at steering sensitivity and linearity as most discriminating factors.

Käppler and Godthelp [6] resulted at reaction accuracy and the amount of steering wheel angle needed as most consistent subjective characteristics. In contrast, they concluded that the number of steering corrections needed as well as the required steering moment show large variation in driver rating, and therefore should be regarded as more individual assessment.

Finally, Mimuro et. al. [9] gave an interpretation of the "rhombus-parameters" in figure 4:

G_r : handling easiness
ω_n : heading responsiveness
ξ_r : directional damping
ϕ : following controllability

2.4. MATCHING TYRE CHARACTERISTICS TO VEHICLE PERFORMANCE

In this subsection, the major conclusions are listed from the references mentioned earlier, based on the classification of table 1.

Differences in tread compound with respect to hardness and hysteresis are well discriminated by the vehicle steering response, indicating how quickly the tyre reacts to a steering input (including both time response and gain). Very low discrimination is found for tracking (how well does the vehicle maintain its course without driver input) and the controllability of the rear end or front end of the car. This result is supported by [6] where it was concluded that different tyre characteristics due to tyre pressure variations have hardly any effect on lateral deviation in straight lane driving.

Different choices for carcass material and belt material yield mixed effects with respect to cornering stiffness, with relative variation in the order of 30 % for the desired conditions. No clear relationship was found in [14]. Increased cornering stiffness is normally associated with a higher yawrate gain and shorter responsetimes, and therefore a better subjective evaluation. This is the reason why radial tyres are preferred above cross-ply tyres. It was shown in [14] that this difference between radial tyres and cross-ply tyres might be counteracted by severe (shoulder) wear-in. In addition, cross-ply tyres were reported to give more "feel" through the steering system [1], explained by the occurrence of a higher pneumatic trail. They show a more linear vehicle response in forward speed making extreme conditions better predictable.

These results do not seem to match with the conclusions by Schröder and Jung (reported in [17]) that the effect of the aligning torque on the handling performance is low. Apparently, "feel" should be interpreted here as something different than handling performance. It might be more related to feedback to the driver through the required steering torque, not effecting gains and response times, and not well covered by objective testmethods presently in use.

There is evidence that cornering stiffness increases with tyre size and reducing aspect ratio. This last observation is consistent with the preference of drivers for low profile radial tyres with respect to steering feel, vehicle stability, road holding and handling. On the other hand, conventional radials are superior to low profile tyres with respect to steering return strength, rural comfort and rural steering performance. Moreover, conventional tyres tend to yield more "linear" behaviour in yawrate and lateral acceleration than low-profile tyres.

Regarding service parameters, some observations are listed below with respect to wet surface conditions, the effect of tyre load and the effect of tyrepressure.
Different sources deal with tests on both dry and wet roads. It was specifically concluded in [14] that wet surface testing is a practical and useful approach for research on vehicle response characteristics. Without getting more specific about this conclusion, it seems to apply to braking tests exclusively. For steering tests, reduced ratings are obtained on wet roads making these wet conditions less suitable for judgement of handling performance.

Tyre loads in general tend to increase the cornering stiffness. The cornering stiffness stabilises beyond a certain load and may even slightly reduce beyond this point. A similar non-linear effect is well-known regarding the inner pressure. A maximum (optimal) cornering stiffness is obtained for a certain pressure with lower values for smaller pressures (deflected tyre) as well as beyond this pressure value (changing contact patch).
The effect of tyre pressure on vehicle handling judgement has been extensively studied in [6] with mixed pressure conditions (different pressure for front and rear tyres) chosen such that three typical understeer-oversteer conditions resulted:
- standard understeer
- extreme understeer (low frontpressure)
- oversteer (low rearpressure)

It was concluded that these tyre pressure variations had hardly any effect on lateral deviation in straight lane driving. In contrast, the required steering activity (magnitude of steering angle as well as the required faster response time) increases with extreme understeer over the entire speed range. A more extreme result was observed in the oversteer situation, however only beyond a certain (critical) speed.

So far, we have considered the impact of changing conditions that refer to the tyre-physics or the service conditions. As mentioned earlier, such variation primarily affect tyre performance parameters and, through these, vehicle performance. Below we will focus directly to these last type of relationships.

As noticed before, a higher cornering stiffness correlates with a better handling evaluation by the driver. One should distinguish here between matched tyre conditions at front and rear, and with mixed tyre characteristics.

A higher cornering stiffness in general leads to lower phase lags both in yaw rate and in lateral acceleration, as well as to a lower phase lag difference between lateral acceleration and yaw rate. In addition, it has been reported to correspond to a lower TB-factor (or "vehicle characteristic") and a higher yaw rate natural frequency.

For mixed conditions, we refer to the comments on [6] and the observation in [14] that

mixed cornering stiffness conditions have impact on the peak lateral acceleration (with trapezoidal steer test, or sinus-steer) indicating a smaller stabilising tolerance (in the sense of figure 2).

Finally, some comments are made on wear-in procedures and normal tyre wear.

It was observed in [14] that the peak lateral force coefficient is strongly effected by tyre shoulder wear, with opposite results for radials and cross-ply tyres. It illustrates that one should be careful about wear-in procedures. More results will come available from the TIME project, the results of which will be published in due time.

The evaluation of the understeer-oversteer characteristics of certain mixed tyrepressure conditions as reported in [6] were repeated after one year of normal use. These characteristics appeared to have developed into a more pronounced direction, both for the pressure combination with original understeer performance and the pressure combination with original oversteer characteristics.

3. THE VARIATION OF TYRE CHARACTERISTICS, A MODEL   APPROACH

The previous section discussed variation in physical tyre parameters, their effect on tyre performance characteristics and their sensitivity with respect to assessment of vehicle performance. Both links, between tyre design and tyre performance as well as between tyre performance and vehicle performance, are still not well understood.

Tyre performance characteristics can be described using the well known Magic Formula tyremodel, the latest version of which for passenger car tyres is described in [12].

Its basic form is given by

$$Y(x) = D.\{\sin \; or \cos\}\left[C \arctan\big(Bx - E(Bx - \arctan(Bx))\big)\right] \qquad (1)$$

with $Y(x)$ equals either brake force (or driving force) or lateral force in case of the sine version, whereas $Y(x)$ is related to the pneumatic trail in case of the cosine version. The variable x denotes the longitudinal or lateral slip. The coefficients B, C, D and E are usually described as stiffness factor, shape factor, peak value and curvature factor, respectively.

In order to study the effect of changing of these characteristics on vehicle handling, various User Scaling Factors have been included in the Magic Formula model. Some of these User Scaling Factors are listed below (restricted here to lateral pure slip):

λ_{Fz0} : nominal load

$\lambda_{\mu y}$: peak friction coefficient

λ_{Ky} : cornering stiffness

λ_{Cy} : shape factor

λ_{Ey} : curvature factor

λ_{yy} : camber force stiffness

λ_{t} : pneumatic trail

For further clarification of these scaling factors, some of the Magic Formula expressions for pure lateral slip are included in (2) - (7). In (2), expressions of the lateral force and aligning torque are given in general terms, depending on wheel position (expressed by slip angle α, camber angle γ), load F_z, pneumatic trail t and residual torque M_{zr}.

$$F_y = F_{y0}(\alpha,\gamma,F_z) \;, \qquad\qquad M_z = M_{z0}(\alpha,\gamma,F_z) = -t.F_{y0} + M_{zr} \qquad (2)$$

The expression (1) is made more explicit in (3), with horizontal and vertical shifts included (absent in (1)) and with the coefficients and their relationship with the scalar factors further clarified (in terms of the tyre load F_z and nominal load F_{z0}). The scalar factor for the pneumatic trail is explained by (7).

$$F_{y0} = D.\sin\left[\arctan\big\{B.\alpha_y - E.\big(B.\alpha_y - \arctan(B.\alpha_y)\big)\big\}\right] + S_V, \; \alpha_y = \alpha + S_H \qquad (3)$$

$$\gamma_y = \gamma.\lambda_{yy} \qquad\qquad\qquad\qquad\qquad\qquad (4)$$

$$D = \mu_y . F_z \ , \quad \mu_y = \mu\left(F_z, \gamma_y\right) . \lambda_{\mu y} \tag{5}$$

$$B = K_y / (C.D), \qquad K_y = K\left(F_z, F_{z0} . \lambda_{Fz0}, \gamma_y\right) . F_{z0} . \lambda_{Fz0} . \lambda_{Ky} \tag{6}$$

$$t(\alpha + S_{Ht}) = t_0\left(\alpha + S_{Ht}\right) . \lambda_t \tag{7}$$

Plots for the side force and pneumatic trail are shown in figures 5 and 6 for varying scalar factors $(\lambda_{Ky}, \lambda_{\mu y})$ (i.e. varying stiffness and friction) and $(\lambda_{Ky}, \lambda_{\mu y}, \lambda_t)$ (i.e. varying stiffness, friction, trail) respectively.

Each scalar factor is chosen from two extreme values, high (indicated with **h**) and low (indicated with **l**).

The scalar factors for cornering stiffness and friction will be varied likewise in the next section in full vehicle simulation studies.

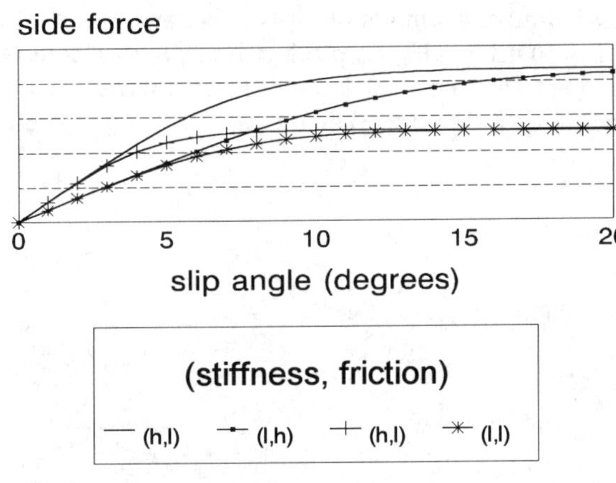

Figure 5.: Side force characteristics

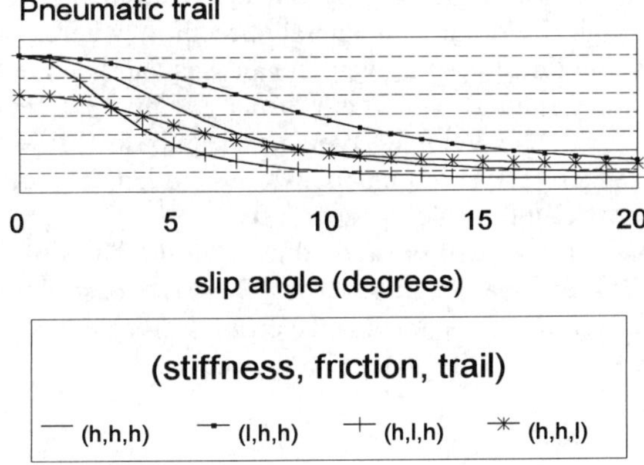

Figure 6.: Pneumatic trail characteristics

4. TYRE SENSITIVITY, SIMULATION STUDIES

In this section, the behaviour of a vehicle under various driving conditions is studied for different values of the cornering stiffness and friction. Two cases are distinguished here, the *"matched case"* with the same characteristics at front and rear tyres, and the *"mixed case"* with different characteristics.

4.1. VARIED TYRE CHARACTERISTICS

For tyres, one of the standard parameter sets is used, contained in MF-TYRE version 5.0 (a subroutine for modelling and simulation of tyre behaviour, based on the Magic Formula, and part of the DELFT-TYRE product line), and related to a passenger car tyre on a dry road. The User Scalar Factors for cornering stiffness and friction are varied according to the following schedule:

$$\lambda_{Ky} \quad : 0.5, 0.6, \ldots, 1.0$$
$$\lambda_{\mu y} \quad : 0.1, 0.2, \ldots, 1.0$$

where the cases mentioned above can be expressed as:

$$\text{matched case}: \lambda_{front} = \lambda_{rear}$$
$$\text{mixed case} \quad : \lambda_{front} \neq \lambda_{rear}$$

4.2. MODELDESCRIPTION AND SELECTED REFERENCE MANOEUVRES

A non-linear vehicle multi-body model has been used in this study with the sprung mass modelled as one (6 dof) rigid body, connected to the unsprung mass with linear springs and dampers. Additional roll stiffness (stabiliser) was included. The tyres were described by the Magical Formula in lateral direction, whereas the vertical behaviour was described by linear springs. The model was validated in the time domain by comparison (and tuning) with data from a complete set of reference handling manoeuvres from the Vehicle Dynamics Database [7] for an existing high performance passenger car. These manoeuvres included the double lane change, the step steer response and the random steer test.

The impact of varying tyre characteristics will be studied here on the basis of two types of steering input tests: the step steer input test (or J-Turn) to describe the response characteristics of the vehicle to a sudden steerinput (response time, overshoot value,...) and the random steer test to generate frequency response data (gain, phase lag,..).

4.3. RESULTS AND INTERPRETATION

Simulations have been carried out for varying cornering stiffness for both the matched and mixed cases, as indicated above. The results are included in annexes 1 and 2.

First, the transferfunctions have been determined. The simulations in the time domain have been carried out for a ramp steer input (approximating the step steer input), growing from 0 to a maximum value within 0.4 sec's, such that a steady state lateral acceleration of 4 m/s^2 was obtained. With an initial speed of 20 m/s, this corresponds to a steady state bend with radius of 100 m.

Lowering the cornering stiffness simultaneously at front and rear tyres leads to lower gain and larger phase lag between steering angle and yaw rate, in contrast to the situation of a reduced lateral stiffness only at the rear tyres. In the latter case, understeer behaviour is reduced and possible oversteer behaviour may result which leads to increased gain at lower frequencies.

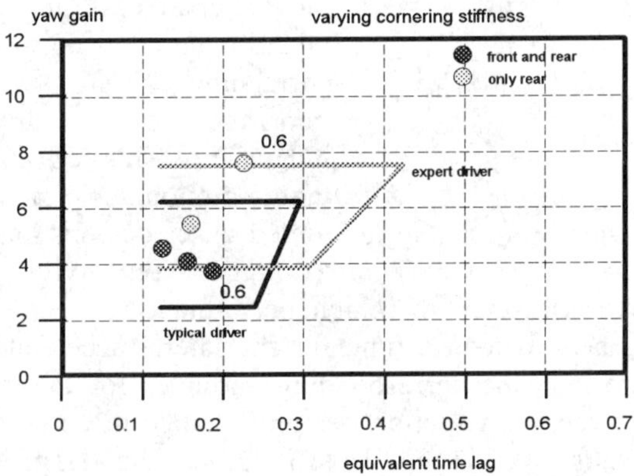

Figure 7.: Comparison with optimal handling boundaries cf. [16]

These results have been included in a "Weir and DiMarco plot, figure 7 similar to figure 3. Lowering cornering stiffness yields a tendency to "leave" the optimal area for both the matched and the mixed case. In the matched case however, this is due to a required larger steering angle whereas the car responds too violently in the mixed case. In both cases, the large equivalent time lag indicates a slower response to steering input.

A stronger steering input (matched case) results into a stronger overshoot as reflected in the time response for the yaw rate in annex 1. Clearly, the contrary is obtained in the mixed case (annex 2) where in both cases the larger response times are evident. Likewise, a similar effect is obtained for the body slipangle. The roll angle is very much associated to the lateral acceleration and doesn't show a very significant difference between the matched and the mixed case.

The various performance indicators, relating to response time, are shown in figures 8 and 9 for different values of the cornering stiffness scaling factor λ_{Ky} for the matched case and mixed case, respectively. Distinction is made between the response time T_x and peak response time $T_{r.\max}$, corresponding to the time from the steering ramp until 90 % of the steady state value or until the maximum value of variable x is reached, respectively.

The variable x indicates yaw rate or lateral acceleration. These times differ in the sense that the stabilising capacity of the car and tyres effects the peak response time. In addition, the time lag between lateral acceleration and yaw rate is shown, as well as the TB factor (vehicle characteristic).

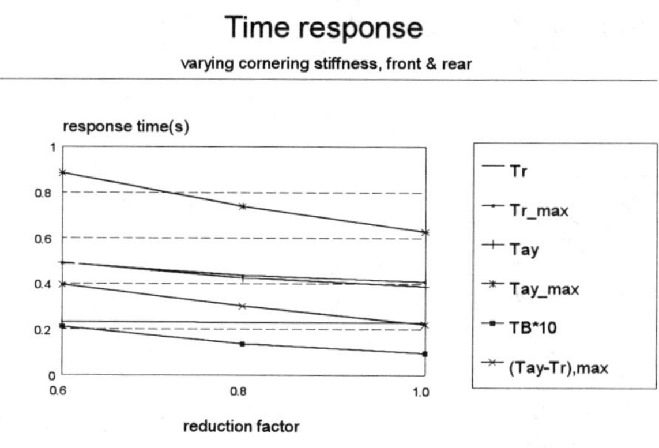

Figure 8.: Time response indicators, matched case

It is interesting to examine the amount of distinction between the three values for the scalar factors, by each of the indicators. Each of the indicators is decreasing with higher cornering stiffness (both in the matched case and the mixed case), normally correlating with an improved driver judgement. This effect is more pronounced in the mixed case, demonstrating a higher sensitivity of cornering stiffness to the subjective assessment of vehicle performance.

However, the response time and peak response time for the lateral acceleration appear to discriminate better here than the corresponding variables for the yaw rate, if one compares the average relative variation per unit change in cornering stiffness. This confirms the results by Xia et al. [17]. Also, the TB-factor distinguishes well between the different values of cornering stiffness and especially the time lag between lateral acceleration and yaw rate shows a good discrimination in both cases.

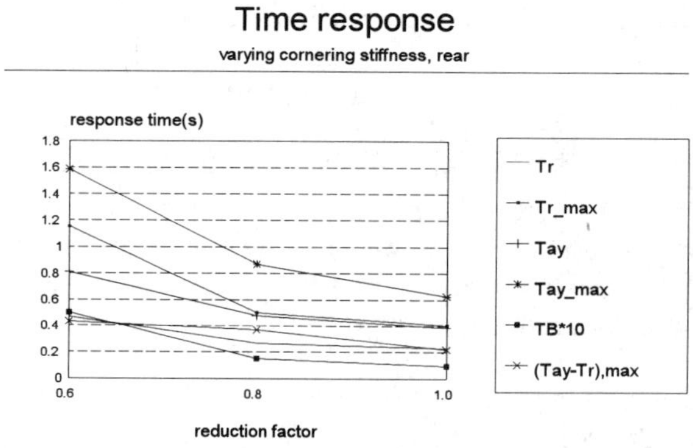

Next, we have varied the friction levels at front and rear tyres independently. As a result, similar conclusions can be derived regarding the resulting response

Figure 9.: Time response indicators, mixed case

times, phase lags, gains, etc. A friction level at the rear tyres, exceeded by the friction at front tyres might yield unstable behaviour, that is, the vehicle shows strong oversteer behaviour and high absolute body slipangles are found.

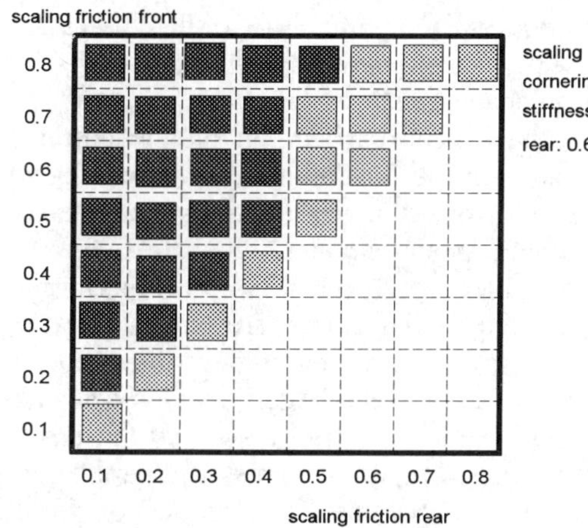

For illustration, the combined effect of reduced cornering stiffness at the rear ($\lambda_{Ky}=0.6$) and mixed friction levels at front and rear is shown in figure 10, where dark squares indicate unstable behaviour. Restoring the cornering stiffness at the rear to the original value ($\lambda_{Ky}=1.0$) slightly improves the stability, but the road friction remains to be the dominant factor.

Figure 10.: Stability under the combined effect of reduced   friction and modified cornering stiffness at the rear.

5. DISCUSSION AND FOLLOW-UP

Various studies on the assessment of vehicle performance have been reviewed, especially related to tyre characteristics. In most cases, this assessment is related to indicators that can be well defined by reference manoeuvres such as J-turn, random steer etc. Parameters such as gains, response times and phase lags are able to distinguish well between certain different tyre performance characteristics. Other tyre characteristics such as pneumatic trail do not result in such clear distinction whereas it was discussed in section 2.4 that a higher pneumatic trail might contribute to a better "feel" through the steering wheel to the driver. Moreover, there is some evidence that the ranking over tyres according to this "feel" does not match the ranking according to the conventional objective indicators such as response times, gains, etc. Another intriguing indicator in this respect is linearity.

We concluded that there might be more impact of tyre performance to the driver assessment and performance then what can be described by the present reference manoeuvres. These observations are confirmed by other sources from which it is known that relatively minor changes in tyre design and tyre characteristics may result in significant dissimilarities in subjective driver assessment. Within the limits of human assessment, to a large extent these driver assessments appear to be reproducible. Dominating tyre properties and, additionally, the highly sensitive vehicle suspension/steering system contribute significantly to this assessment-reproducibility. However, it is presently insufficiently clear how such driver judgements are related to vehicle design characteristics.

Many of the studies reviewed above have been carried out on the correlation between driver ratings and objective assessments for dominant vehicle behaviour. However, the situation may be more involved than situations considered in previous studies. It means that relatively small parameter deviations yet have significant influence. Methods to objectively quantify the performance deterioration due to these small parameter deviations are virtually lacking. Further, it is not understood how results of such newly developed objective assessment methods could assist in improving the vehicle design. This demands to develop insight into the information available to and criteria used by the driver in his judgement process, and into their relation with key variables and parameters of the vehicle. Identifying these key variables and parameters in connection with the information transferred through these variables to the driver constitutes a main research issue, yet to be undertaken.

6. CONCLUSIONS

Tyres have a strong impact on driver judgement of vehicle performance. In addition, the tyre-road interface constitutes a critical factor in the risk reduction potential at critical situations. Due to the interaction of tyre response with other vehicle subsystems (suspension, steering), it is however difficult to obtain a clear understanding of this impact.

Some previous studies have been reviewed, focusing on a large variety of input tyre characteristics, methodologies (reference tests, subjective ratings, etc.) and performance metrics such as gains, time lags, special indicators such as the TB-factor. Input variables could be connected to tyre construction, tyre geometry or dimensions, service parameters such as inner pressure, ageing, etc.

Some authors exploit combinations of these indicators to obtain a broader view of the vehicle performance. It is apparent that a large variety of input and output parameters as well as test procedures exist, where more standard test procedures and subjective factors would be preferred.

Using the scaling options in DELFT-TYRE, simulation studies have been carried out for a realistic and validated vehicle model under random steer and step steer loading. Differences in tyre characteristics are well distinguished by many of the vehicle objective performance indicators discussed earlier.

Summarising, the understanding of the impact of tyre characteristics on driver assessment is limited and deserves further attention. This requires more sophisticated tools, both with reference to simulation and experiments. There is a need for new objective testmethods and more standardisation in the subjective rating scheme, where distinction should be made between normal conditions and emergency situations.

ACKNOWLEDGEMENTS

I am grateful to Sven Jansen for his valuable contribution in the preparations of the simulation model.

REFERENCES

[1]   BRINDLE, L.R., WILSON, W.T.: The Effects of Tyre Type on Driver Perception and Risk-Taking. International Conference of Vehicle Handling. Institute of Mechanical Engineers C134/83, London (1983)

[2]   BRINDLE, L.R.: The Influence of Tyre Characteristics on Driver Opinion. Applied Psychology Executive Report. Cranfield Institute of Technology (1984).

[3]   DONGES, E.: Supporting Drivers by Chassis Control Systems. In.: PAUWELUSSEN J.P., PACEJKA, H.B.: Smart Vehicles. Swets & Zeitlinger Publishers (1995).

[4]   FAIRLIE, A.M., POTTINGER M.G.: Statistics of Double Lane Change Handling Tests Conducted on Tires Differing in Tread Compound Physical Properties. SAE Technical Paper Series 880583 (1983)

[5]   RANDWIJK, M.J. v., GODTHELP, J., KÄPPLER, M.W.D., RUIJS, P.A.J.: Correlation of Driver Judgement and Vehicle Directional Data to Evaluate and Predict Truck Handling. Third EAEC Conference, Strassbourg, France (1991)

[6]   KÄPPLER, W-D., GODTHELP, J.: The Effects of Tire Pressure Variations on Vehicle Handling Properties and Driving Strategy. Forschung für Anthropotechnik, Bericht Nr. 72 (1986)

[7]   KÄPPLER, W-D., GODTHELP, J., RANDWIJK, M.J.v., RUIJS, P.A.J.: Methodology for Predicting Car and Truck Handling Assessments. Institute of Mechanical Engineers C389/379 (1992)

[8]   KLEUSKENS, R.J.A..: The TNO Vehicle Dynamics Database (VDD). A Tool for Comparison of Vehicles Dynamics Behaviour. Autotest '96, IDIADA Spain (1996)

[9]   MIMURO, T. et.al.: Four Parameter Evaluation Method of Lateral Transient Response. SAE Paper 901734 (1990)

[10] OOSTEN, J.J.M.v., BAKKER, E.: Determination of Magic Formula Tyre

Model Parameters. Proceedings 1st International Colloquium on Tyre Models for Vehicle Dynamic Analysis.
Swets & Zeitlinger B.V., Amsterdam/Lisse (1993).

[11]   PACEJKA, H.B.: The Role of Tyre Dynamic Properties.
In.: PAUWELUSSEN J.P., PACEJKA, H.B.: Smart Vehicles. Swets & Zeitlinger Publishers (1995).

[12]   PACEJKA, H.B.: The Tyre as a Vehicle Component.
XXVI FISITA Congress Prague (1996)

[13]   J.P. PAUWELUSSEN: Assessment of Traffic Safety Margin in Adverse Weather Conditions. In.: KROES, J.L. de, STOOP, J.A.: First World Congress on Transport Safety, Delft (1992)

[14]   ROLAND, R.D., RICE, R.S., DELL'AMICO, F.: The Influence of Tire Properties on Passenger Vehicle Handling. Calspan Corporation Report (1975)

[15]   SAVKOOR, A., HAPPEL, H., HORKAY, F.: Vehicle Transient Response to Steering Input. In.: PAUWELUSSEN J.P.: Understanding Human Monitoring and Assessment. Swets & Zeitlinger Publishers (1995).

[16]   WEIR, D.H., DIMARCO, R.J.: Correlation and Evaluation of Driver/Vehicle Directional Handling Data. SAE Paper 780010 (1978)

[17]   XIA, X., WILLIS, J.N., The Effects of Tire Cornering Stiffness on Vehicle Linear Handling Performance.
SAE Technical Paper Series 950313 (1995)

ANNEX 1.: VARYING CORNERING STIFFNESS, MATCHED CASE.

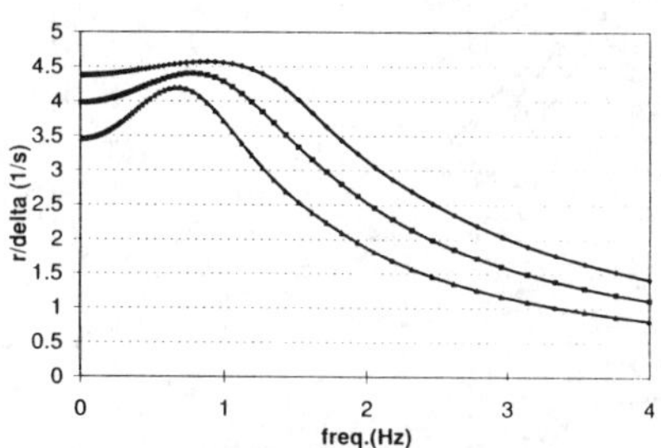

Fig. A1.: Yaw rate transfer function, gain.
$\lambda_{Ky} = 1.0, 0.8, 0.6$ (top down)
front and rear

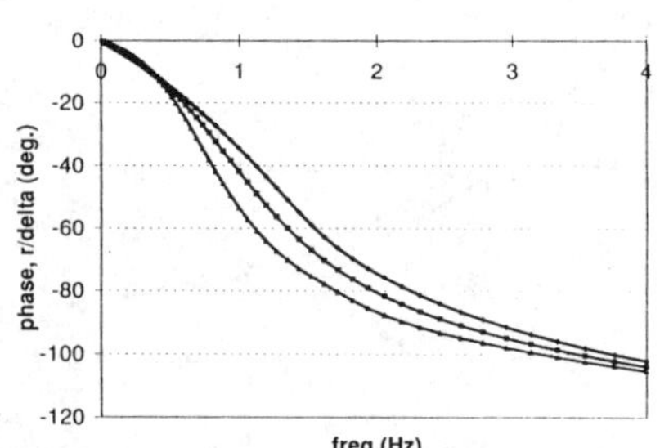

Fig. A2.: Yaw rate gain transfer function, phase lag
$\lambda_{Ky} = 1.0, 0.8, 0.6$ (top down)
front and rear

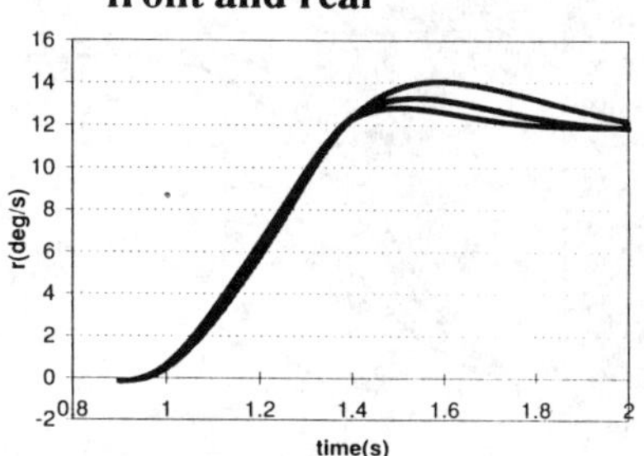

Fig. A3.: Yaw rate time response
$\lambda_{Ky} = 1.0, 0.8, 0.6$ (bottom up)
front and rear

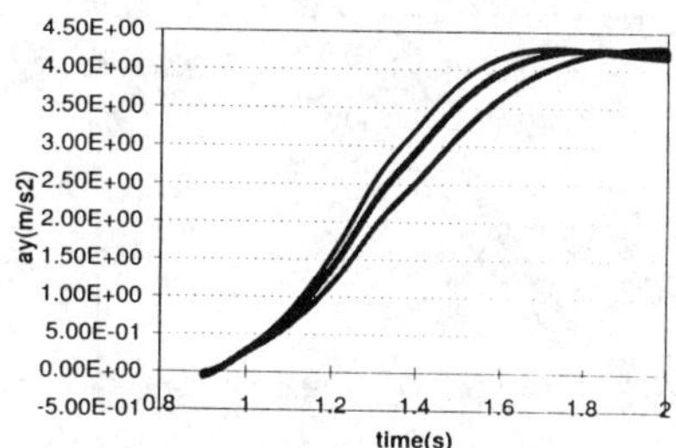

Fig. A4.: Lateral accel. time response
$\lambda_{Ky} = 1.0, 0.8, 0.6$ (top down)
front and rear

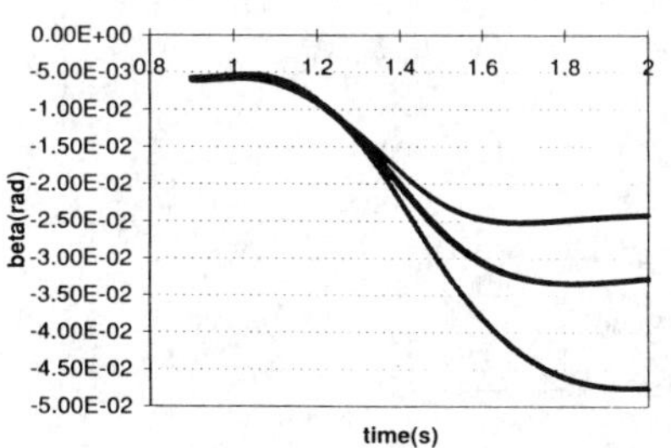

Fig. A5.: Body slipangle time resp.
$\lambda_{Ky} = 1.0, 0.8, 0.6$ (top down)
front and rear

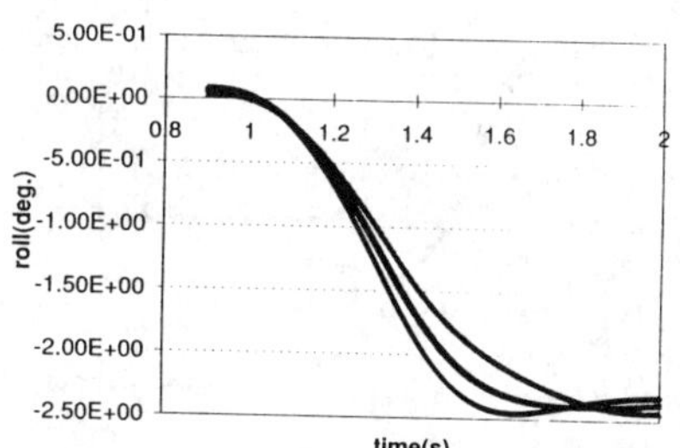

Fig. A6.: Roll angle time response
$\lambda_{Ky} = 1.0, 0.8, 0.6$ (bottom up)
front and rear

ANNEX 2.: VARYING CORNERING STIFFNESS, MIXED CASE.

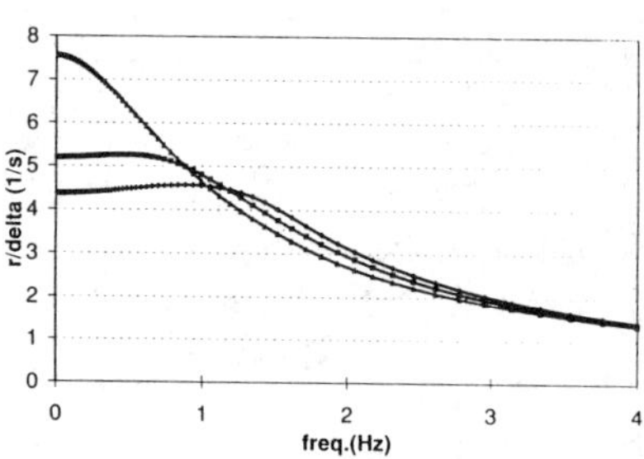

Fig. A7.: Yaw rate transfer function, gain.
λ_{Ky} = 1.0, 0.8, 0.6 (bottum up)
only rear

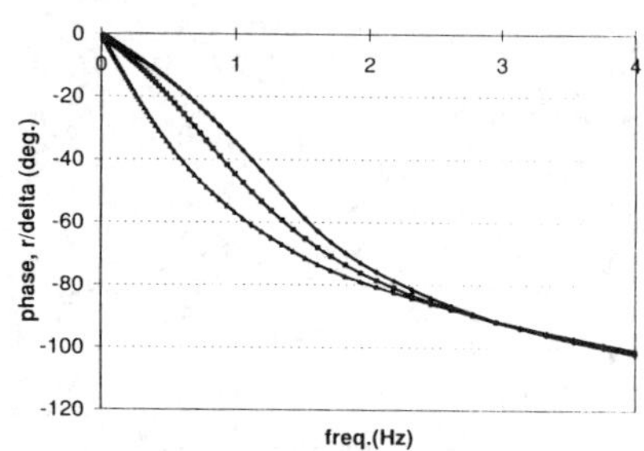

Fig. A8.: Yaw rate gain transfer function, phase lag
λ_{Ky} = 1.0, 0.8, 0.6 (top down)
only rear

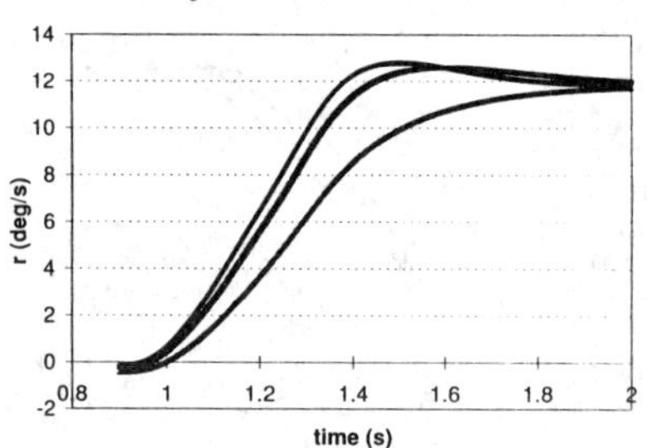

Fig. A9.: Yaw rate time response
λ_{Ky} = 1.0, 0.8, 0.6 (top down)
only rear

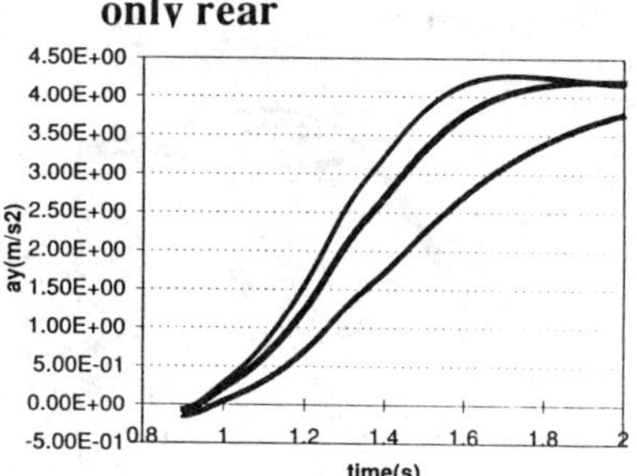

Fig. A10.: Lateral accel. time response
λ_{Ky} = 1.0, 0.8, 0.6 (top down)
only rear

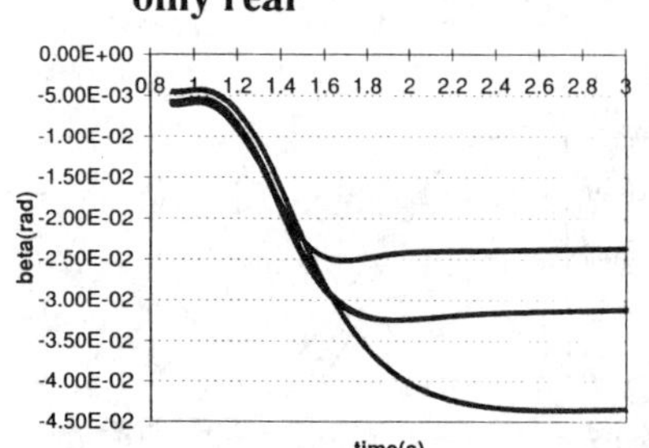

Fig. A11.: Body slipangle time resp.
λ_{Ky} = 1.0, 0.8, 0.6 (top down)
only rear

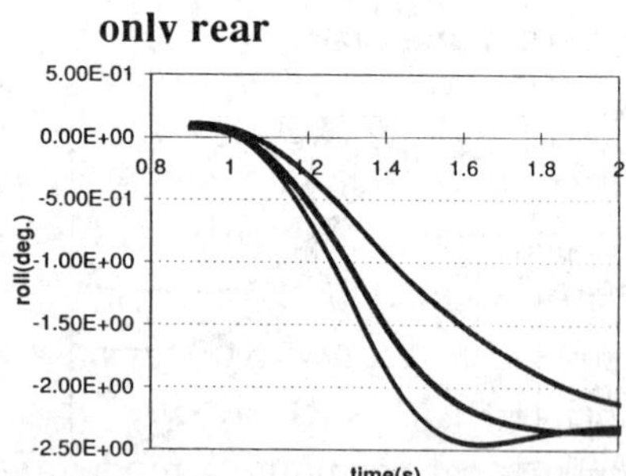

Fig. A12.: Roll angle time response
λ_{Ky} = 1.0, 0.8, 0.6 (bottom up)
only rear

Vehicle Performance: J.P. Pauwelussen (ed.) pp. 177-195

INFLUENCE OF THE TYRE ON SUBJECTIVE HANDLING AT THE LIMIT

P Stephens

H J Kohn

A brief description is given of the force and moment generation properties of tyres, and the methods available for measuring them. Simple tyre parameters may be derived from these measurements and used by tyre engineers to estimate the handling performance of vehicles. Problems associated with such a 'tyre only approach' are discussed. The use of mathematical (computer) modelling techniques can be used to overcome many of these problems. However, the tyre designer is still required to interpret the objective data from the model in terms of subjective ratings used by test drivers. Finally, two mathematical models, developed as part of a joint project between Dunlop Tyres, Department of Transport (UK), and Jaguar/Ford, are described, together with handling parameters relateable to subjective limit handling assessment.

1. INTRODUCTION

Tyres generate the principal forces and moments which govern a vehicle's handling characteristics. Tyre lateral force, created by slip and camber mechanisms is responsible for cornering, while aligning torque produced by the vehicle's front tyres contributes to handwheel feel. The tyre's vertical stiffness affects the vehicle's roll behaviour. In addition most tyres produce an audible warning as the friction limit is approached.

2. OBTAINING TYRE DATA AT DUNLOP TYRES LTD.

Accurate tyre data is difficult and expensive to acquire. Experimentally it can be obtained using specialised indoor test machines or by using instrumented trailers, operating on real road surfaces.

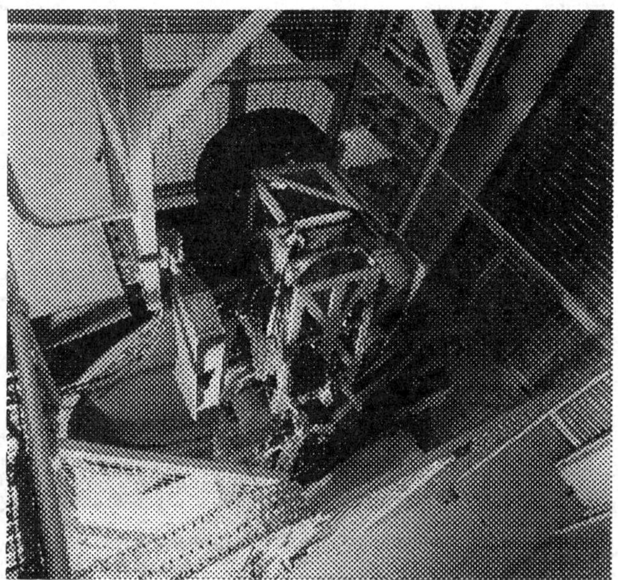

fig1

For car tyre work, Dunlop Ltd. has the Car Tyre Dynamics Machine. This indoor facility was developed in house, and is shown in figure 1. It consists of a 2.39m diameter cast iron drum and a tyre suspension system. The drum is usually surfaced with a coarse textured, high friction material (Resin Bond™) and may be driven at speeds of up to 220 kph. The tyre suspension unit is capable of steering the tyre with respect to the drum surface to obtain slip angles of up to 14°. The tyre may also be tilted with respect to the vertical plane to achieve camber angles of up to 14°. Tyre load may be varied up to approximately 800 kgf. Tyre generated forces and moments are measured by a strain gauged cube, mounted behind the hub. These values are used to compute the forces and moments at the origin of the SAE J670e axis system, (nominally the centre of the tyre's contact patch.) as shown in figure 2. SAE J670e sign conventions are also used. Tyre testing can be carried out under steady state, pseudo steady state and dynamic conditions.

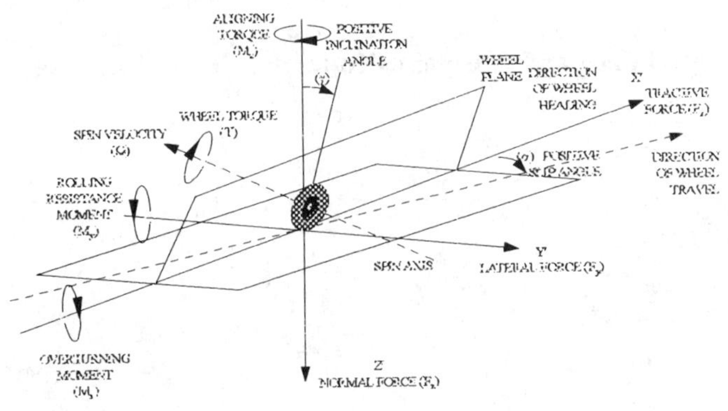

fig 2

Data obtained from indoor test machines should be used with caution. Road surfaces vary in texture and friction properties and it is almost impossible for an indoor test system to duplicate any particular tyre/road combination exactly. Care is required to minimise tyre wear which can substantially increase the effective shear stiffness of the tyre tread region. Tread wear is likely to be a severe problem in obtaining tyre properties appropriate to limit handling. Additionally, for drum machines, curvature of the contact patch is likely to have a small, unpredictable, effect on tyre cornering properties[1].

The biggest limitation of the Car Tyre Dynamics Machine is its inability to test under conditions of longitudinal slip. However, Dunlop Ltd. has access to MTS Flat Trac® test machines within the SRI Group which have this facility.

In addition to physically measuring tyre cornering characteristics, Dunlop Tyres Ltd uses a sophisticated beam on an elastic support mathematical tyre model (TPP -Tyre Property Prediction) to calculate tyre properties from the tyre's geometry (input as a meshed section) and the mechanical properties of the materials used in its construction[2]. Finite element analysis is currently under investigation as a possible alternative method of calculating cornering properties. At present the TPP program is unable to predict accurately the performance of a tyre subjected to combined slip and camber due to its relatively simple friction model, and finite element modelling suffers from long run times. However, modelling is especially useful at the tyre development stage, since it allows tyre properties to be estimated without the cost and effort required to produce moulds. Further advances are expected in this area.

3. TYPICAL TYRE PROPERTIES

Steady State Force and Moment Properties due to Slip Angle

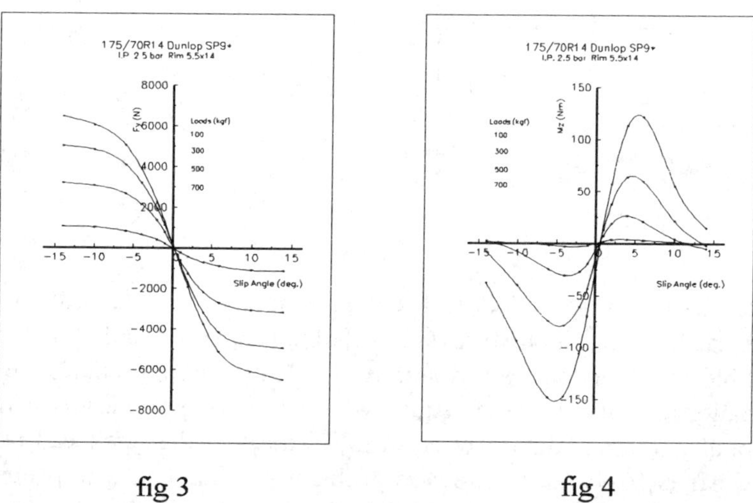

fig 3	fig 4

Figures 3 and 4 show a set of typical force and moment results obtained from the Dunlop Car Tyre Dynamics Machine.

The Lateral Force v Slip Angle graphs show a characteristic shape. At low slip angles the curves are linear with a slope related to the tyre's stiffness properties and contact patch area. At larger slip angles there is a transition region where the slope decreases until it approaches the zero or reversed slope of the saturated tyre. At saturation, the sideforce becomes dependent on the frictional properties of the tyre / road interface.

Aligning torque is more non-linear with slip angle, showing a pronounced peak after the linear low slip angle region and falling to zero as the lateral force graph approaches saturation. The direction of the slip angle aligning torque is predominantly to steer the tyre in a direction to reduce the slip angle and hence the lateral force generated.

Both lateral force and aligning torque are sensitive to load. Increasing the vertical load on the tyre increases both the low slip angle slope and the saturation/peak value of the graphs. In the case of the lateral force graphs,

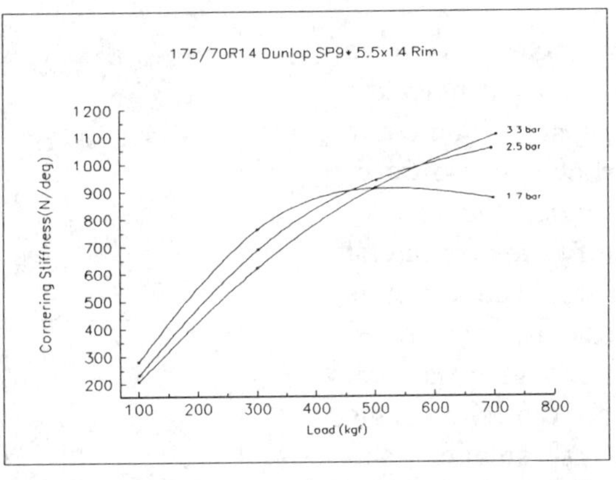

fig 5

the lateral coefficient of friction decreases slightly with increasing load and inflation pressure. The low slip angle slope (cornering stiffness) initially increases with load as the size of the tyre contact patch increases. At higher loads, the rate of increase in cornering stiffness reduces. At very high loads, cornering stiffness may even decrease, due to buckling of the overloaded tyre structure. Increasing inflation pressure both reduces the contact patch area and stabilises the tyre structure in overload conditions. This produces the crossover in the effect of inflation pressure on cornering stiffness shown in figure 5. Cornering Stiffness is decreased by increasing inflation pressure at low loads and increased by increasing inflation pressure at high loads. In dry conditions increasing inflation pressure reduces the effective lateral friction slightly. In wet conditions the higher contact pressure produced by increasing the inflation pressure may increase friction by squeezing water out of the contact patch.

Camber

Cambering a radial tyre with respect to the road surface produces both a lateral force (camber thrust) and an 'aligning' torque. Compared with slip angle generated lateral force, that produced by camber is about 15 - 25 times smaller for an equivalent angle. In the range of cambers normally experienced by a car tyre both camber thrust and camber aligning torque are linear with camber angle. Both are sensitive to load changes. In contrast to slip angle aligning torque, camber aligning torque acts in a direction that tends to steer the tyre to increase the lateral force generated by the camber mechanism.

Combined Slip and Camber Angle

At small slip angles the main effect of camber is to displace the cornering force v slip angle curve vertically, as shown in figure 6. At large slip angles the camber appears to modify the tyre lateral friction properties. The effect is most easily seen at high loads. Where the camber angle is such as to reinforce the slip angle lateral force at smaller slip angles, lateral friction tends to be increased, and vice versa. The changes in friction are not symmetrical. The loss in friction generally outweighs the gain.

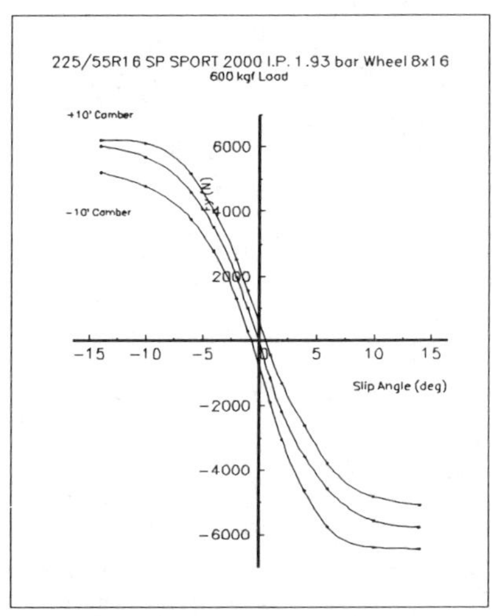

fig 6

Some data obtained using the SRI Flat Trac machine indicate that these results may be reversed at low loads.

Longitudinal Slip

Longitudinal slip produces longitudinal accelerating and braking forces. At small slip angles, lateral force is not sensitive to moderate levels of longitudinal force generation. At high slip angles, the simultaneous application of longitudinal and lateral slip results in a significant decrease in cornering force. This is shown in figure 7. The behaviour of aligning torque under these conditions is complex, often involving sign changes as longitudinal slip is varied.

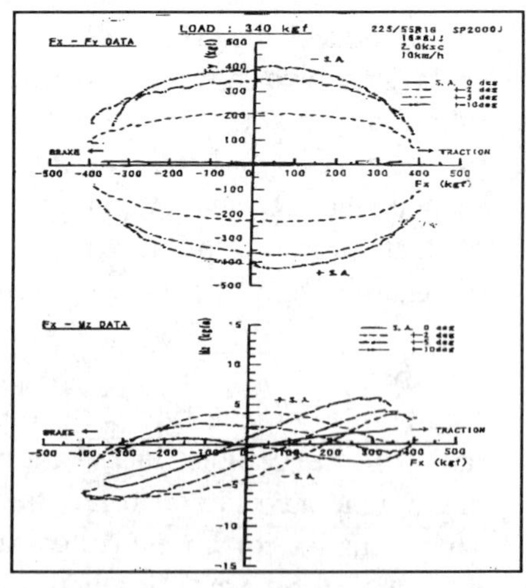

fig 7

Time Dependence

Tyre cornering force is not generated the instant slip angle is applied. If a step steer input is applied to a tyre, cornering force rises exponentially to a steady state value. The level of sideforce after the application of the step steering input is related to the distance the tyre has rolled rather than the elapsed time. The dynamic properties of the tyre may be characterised by its relaxation length. This is the distance that the tyre rolls to reach (1 - 1/e) of its steady state cornering force.

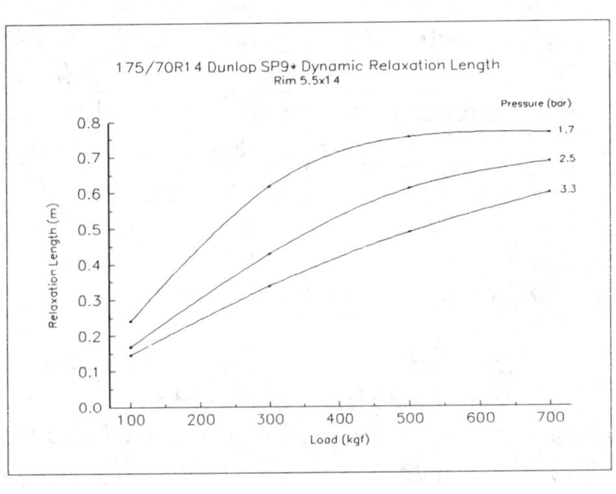

fig 8

Figure 8 illustrates the effect of load and inflation pressure on relaxation length. Increasing inflation pressure decreases relaxation length, increasing tyre load increases relaxation length and vice versa. Relaxation length also depends on the slip angle state of the tyre, and decreases with increasing slip angle.

Tyre Handling Parameters

From the basic tyre property measurements a set of parameters related to vehicle handling may be calculated. These are as follows

Parameter	Description
Cornering Stiffness	Absolute value of the slope of the cornering force v slip angle plot at zero slip angle
Aligning Stiffness	Slope of the aligning torque v slip angle plot at zero slip angle
Pneumatic trail	Moment arm at which the cornering force acts with respect to the SAE 670e axis origin
Camber Stiffness	Slope of the camber thrust v camber angle plot at zero camber angle
Parameter	Description

Camber Aligning Stiffness	Slope of the camber aligning torque v camber angle plot at zero camber angle
Load Sensitivity[3]	Slope of the cornering stiffness v load plot over a nominal load range.
Load Transfer Sensitivity[3]	A measure of the linearity of the cornering force v load plot at a 4° slip angle at a nominal load
Relaxation length	Distance travelled to reach 63.2% of steady state side force following a step steer input
Gough Plot	Plot of cornering force against aligning torque

4. HANDLING 'RULES OF THUMB'

Over the years many general rules have been used by tyre engineers to relate the tyre parameters of the table to subjective vehicle handling. What follows is by way of example, and not intended to be a complete list.

The tyres should be chosen with cornering stiffnesses which ensure that the vehicle has an understeering cornering characteristic.

High cornering stiffness is considered to be desirable, especially on the rear axle. This reduces the rear tyre slip angle and hence the vehicle slip angle required in the steady state, and thus tends to reduce the vehicle's response times.

Relaxation length has been subjectively related to low severity steering responsiveness, and may influence high severity handling on rough road surfaces.

High values of load sensitivity are associated with operating on the more linear part of the tyre's cornering stiffness/load characteristic. In this region the vehicle's understeer characteristics are less sensitive to changes in vehicle centre of gravity. However, the vehicle is more susceptible to road uneveness.

Load transfer sensitivity is a measure of the loss of cornering force on an axle due to load transfer in a severe corner. It is a measure of the tyres sensitivity to the vehicle's suspension configuration. (Front and rear roll stiffness, and their modification by anti roll bar fitment etc.)

Pneumatic trail, aligning stiffness and Gough plot shape relate directly to the tyre component of steering feel. In particular, Gough plot shape is regarded as a good measure of the tyre's contribution to steering feel in the transition region between severe and limit handling conditions.

Camber stiffness and camber aligning stiffness are related to the vehicles susceptibility to lateral road uneveness ('motorway grooving') and poor suspension kinematics in limit handling manoeuvres.

Although these simple tyre related rules are of use in tyre development, it is not possible to use them to predict the handling behaviour of any particular vehicle. As described above, tyre cornering force generation is sensitive to camber attitude and loading changes and these are a function of vehicle centre of gravity, inertias, and suspension design. In order to combine tyre and vehicle effects some form of mathematical model is required.   This also has the advantage of enabling simulated vehicle handling data to be obtained from theoretical tyre properties produced by TPP or similar programs.

5. VEHICLE HANDLING MODELS

Over the last three years Dunlop Tyres Ltd. has collaborated with Jaguar/Ford and Cranfield University in a project to study the Controllability of ROad Vehicles at the Limit of Adhesion (CROVLA). This has involved the development of two vehicle models. The first model is restricted to steady state manoeuvres, while the second model is designed primarily for non-steady state simulations.

The second model was created using the AUTOSIM™ computer language. This generates computationally efficient simulation programs for multibody systems. The modeller describes the system as a series of LISP statements These are then processed by AUTOSIM™ to produce simulation code, such as FORTRAN code, containing equations defining the behaviour of the system.

The two models have many common features. They have six body degrees of freedom plus one degree for each unsprung mass. Suspension kinematic properties (track change, wheel camber, roll steer etc.) are calculated as low order polynomial functions of wheel travel, which give a good fit to real data. Kinematic steering changes are input as functions of lower steering column rotation. Also accounted for are, body torsional stiffness, steering toe in/out, mechanical trail and steering compliance. Rear wheel steering compliance and camber compliance is not considered. Additionally, the non-steady state AUTOSIM™ model incorporates a simple representation of power assisted steering. The models are designed to be generic. Vehicle parameters are input from a separate file and are easily changeable. For the validation study, a full set of vehicle data for the test car (Jaguar XJ6) was supplied by the manufacturers.

The tyre properties were incorporated into the vehicle models using a tyre model based on the Magic Formula of Pacejka and Bakker as described in 1991[4]. The model was restricted to the free rolling case with no attempt to model longitudinal slip. In addition, it was found that setting the curve shape constant a_0 to 1.0, instead of the suggested 1.3, gave a better fit to cornering force data produced using the Car Tyre Dynamics Machine, which shows virtually no decrease at maximum slip.

6. VEHICLE MODEL VALIDATION

Experimental work was carried out at the Motor Industry Research Association test facilities, using an instrumented Jaguar XJ6 vehicle, to provide test data for simulation validation. The manoeuvres used for validation included steady state cornering, ISO lane change and lane change in a turn.

Steady State Cornering
Figure 9 shows handling diagrams for both models and the actual car. The

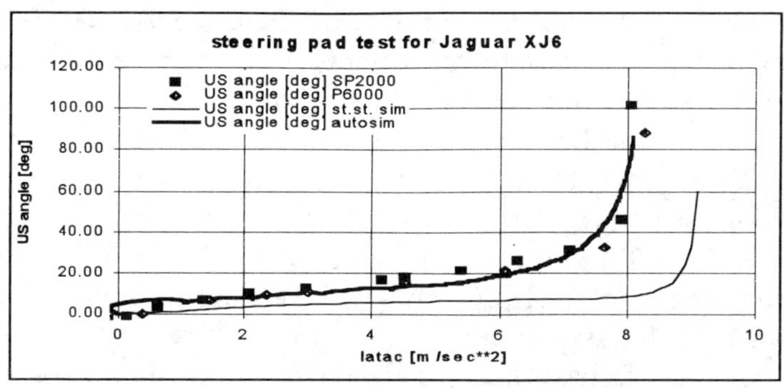

fig 9

understeer angle, the angle which must be added to the Ackermann angle to maintain constant lateral acceleration, is plotted along the horizontal axis. Proving ground results for standard 225/55R16 Dunlop SP2000 test tyres are indicated by squares, while those obtained using a set of part worn Pirelli tyres of the same size are denoted by diamonds. The AUTOSIM™ model results are shown by the thick line, while the Steady State model is indicated by the thin line. Both models use Pacejka model parameters for the Dunlop SP2000 tyre obtained using the Car Tyre Dynamics Machine. The AUTOSIM™ model is in excellent agreement with the experimental measurements, matching the linear behaviour (up to 6 m/s^2), and the transition to limit behaviour. Even the limit lateral acceleration of about 8 m/s^2 was predicted accurately. This is surprising since the tyre data are based on results acquired using the high friction Resin Bond surface.

Figure 10 shows the relationship between steady state lateral acceleration and roll angle found for the models and the real car. Here

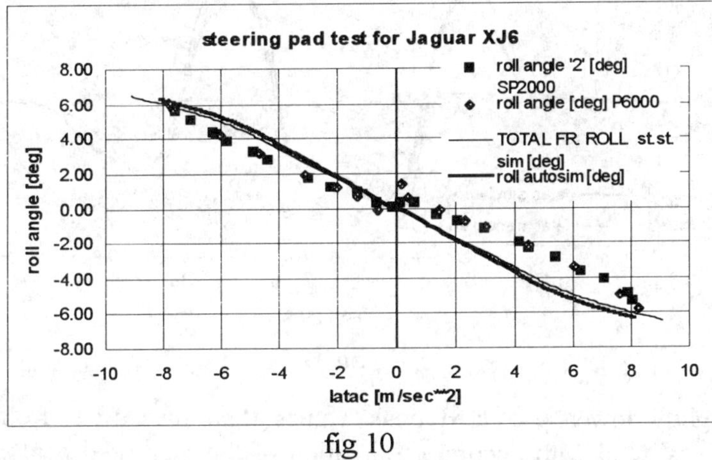

fig 10

agreement is not so good, with the simulation predicting larger roll angles than measured at intermediate lateral accelerations.

Non-Steady State Manoeuvres

Figures 11, 12 and 13 show a comparison of vehicle and model behaviour for a high severity lane change manoeuvre. The simulations were carried

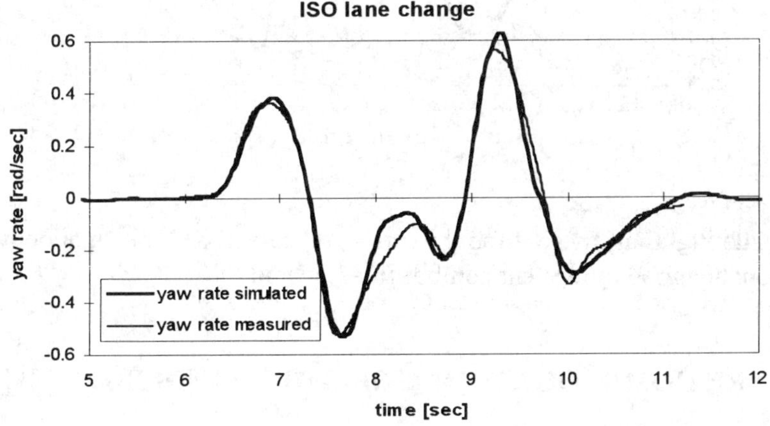

fig 11

out, at constant throttle in open loop mode, by taking the measured vehicle handwheel angle as input. Simulation results are shown as thick lines. A very good match is seen for yaw rate.   Lateral acceleration is less good

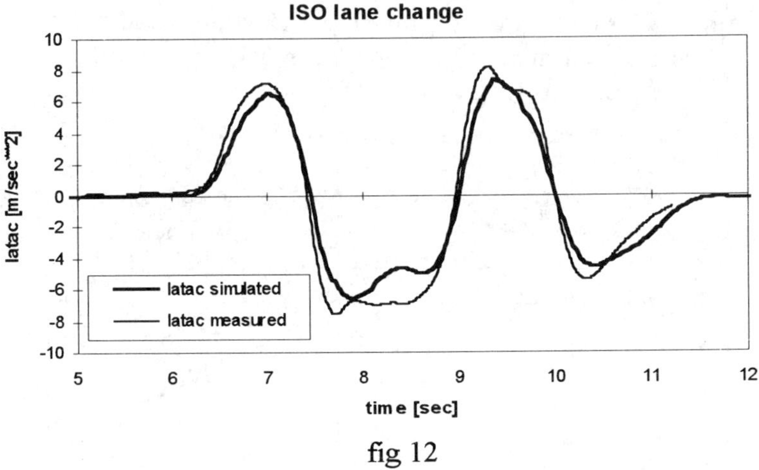

fig 12

with slightly lower predicted peak values than measured. Roll angle matching is good with accurate estimation of the measured peak values.

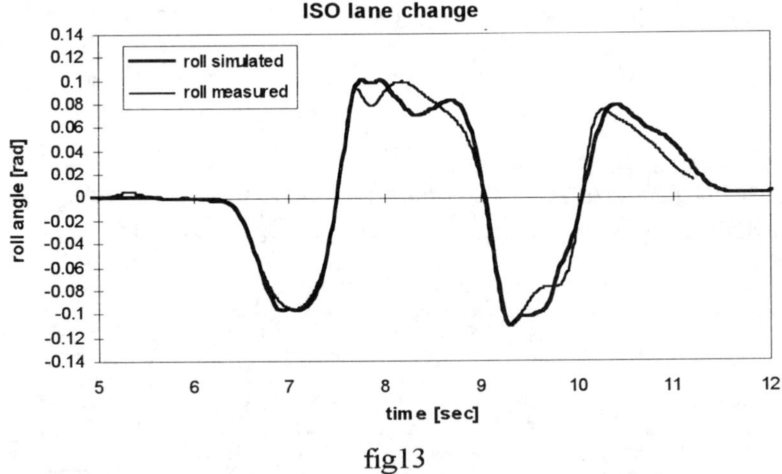

fig13

Considering that these time histories represent a limit manoeuvre, a reasonably good agreement can be stated overall.

7. TYRE HOMOLOGATION AND LIMIT HANDLING QUALITY

In general, handling assessments used in developing new tyres for homologation by vehicle manufacturers are subjective. Each aspect of handling (centre feel, turn in, progression, limit etc.) is normally rated on a numerical scale (typically 1 to 10, though this often becomes compressed). This raises the issue of relating these subjective ratings to the objective handling data available from computer handling simulations. These data are essentially the same as those available from a fully instrumented vehicle.

In limit handling evaluations, significant differences exist between the capabilities of normal drivers and professional test drivers used by both tyre and vehicle manufacturers in tyre homologation studies. The professional driver is capable of keeping a vehicle very close to the tyre saturation limit during a limit handling test. Consequently, the warning factors such as steering weight and tyre squeal, which are normally associated with the initial part of the tyre's linear / saturation transistion region, are not weighted heavily in their limit handling rating. Warning of the vehicle's handling limit is still considered important and this is judged by professional drivers from changes in the vehicle's steering response[5].

Although exact handling requirements vary with manufacturer and vehicle type, some general ideas about handling quality have been developed[6]. Handling a vehicle should be made easy in order to relieve the driver from any tiring control strain. This can be achieved if the vehicle responds to the driver's control commands in a consistent and predictable manner, throughout its operating range, changing progressively as the tyres saturate towards the handling limit. A straight forward relationship between driver control on one hand, and vehicle reaction on the other is desired, which ideally prevails for all conditions, irrespective of surface friction or irregularity.

Vehicle response times have to be regarded as properties relevant in determining handling quality. It is obvious that long reaction times between driver control and vehicle response render a vehicle uncontrollable, especially for high speed manoeuvring, for which a desired position or attitude correction has to be assumed in a short distance of travel. Other research[7,8] indicates that short control delay times seem to constitute a significant benefit for normal driving manoeuvres. Moderately long time lags may be compensated by an appropriate preview strategy. However, short response times are desirable for completing an emergency manoeuvre, for which the emphasis lies on fast closed-loop control.

8. CROSS CORRELATION AS A LIMIT HANDLING PARAMETER

Considering the factors described above, and at the suggestion of Sharp[9], the concept of correlation has been assessed as a handling quality parameter. This technique allows the comparison of the overall shape of two signals and the delay between them.

The same instrumented vehicle as used in the model validation was used to investigate the interaction between the driver perception and vehicle handling for transient manoeuvres, such as lane changes. Handwheel position was found to be the best driver control signal for this manoeuvre. Vehicle response was characterised by its yaw rate, lateral acceleration and roll angle time histories. When the cross-correlation technique is applied to a vehicle control input and response, the correlation coefficient and time delay provide measures of handling quality which are independent of driver skill. The correlation coefficient is calculated from the correlation function $c(\tau)$ defined as:

$$c(\tau) = \frac{\int_0^T x(t) \cdot y(t + \tau)dt}{\sqrt{\int_0^T x(t)^2 dt \cdot \int_0^T y(t)^2 dt}}, \text{ where}$$

$x(t)$ denotes the input signal after removing its mean,

$y(t)$ denotes the output signal after removing its mean,

T denotes the sequence length considered for analysis and

τ denotes the relative time shift between the signals $y(t)$ and $y(t + \tau)$

Here $x(t)$ denotes the handwheel angle signal and $y(t)$ either the vehicle yaw rate or lateral acceleration.

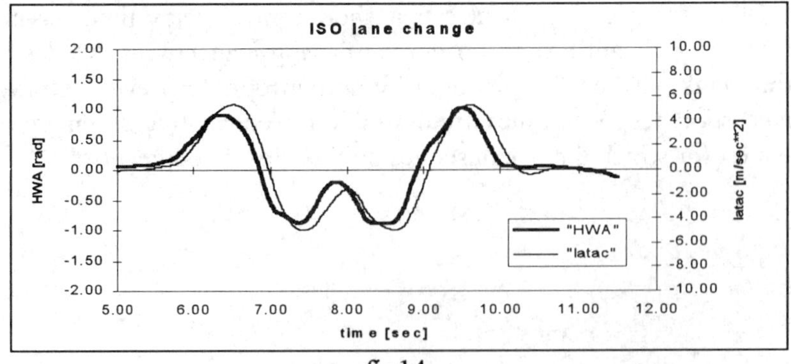

fig14

Figures 14 and 15 illustrate how the idea of correlation can be used to assess the handling of a vehicle. They show handwheel angle and lateral acceleration time histories for the ISO lane change, conducted at speeds of 21 m/s and 27 m/s (the highest speed at which the manoeuvre could be successfully performed). At the lower speed, the test driver was able to perform the manoeuvre with no difficulty whatsoever. Here, the handwheel angle and lateral acceleration response are closely matched. At the higher speed, where the driver experienced considerable difficulty in performing the test, the lateral acceleration time history is a shifted, significantly more

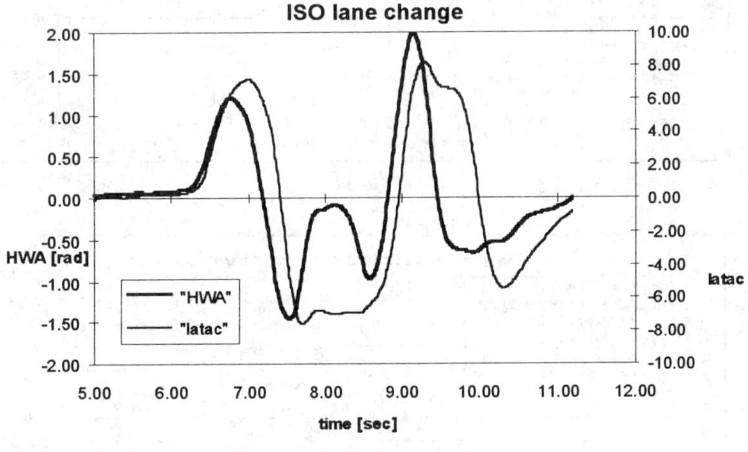

fig15

distorted, image of the handwheel input, resulting in a lower correlation coefficient and increased delay.

9. CROSS-CORRELATION AND SUBJECTIVE ASSESSMENT

A small amount of experimental work has been carried out to relate correlation coefficient and time lag calculated from measurements obtained using the Jaguar instrumented vehicle to subjective driver assessments. Both tyre and vehicle variations were investigated.

Tyres
Three tyre types were evaluated;

[m/s²]

Dunlop SP2000J	225/55R16	Standard Production
Dunlop M2	225/60R16	Winter Pattern
Dunlop XY		Plain Tread Experimental

Subjectively the limit handling of these tyres is rated, from worst to best, in the order M2, SP2000J, XY. Results are compared in figures 16 and 17. Points represented by filled markers indicate tests for which the throttle was held almost constant, whereas their unfilled counterparts denote those for which the standard deviation of the throttle position signal exceeded a threshold value of 20% of its mean. Standard tyres are

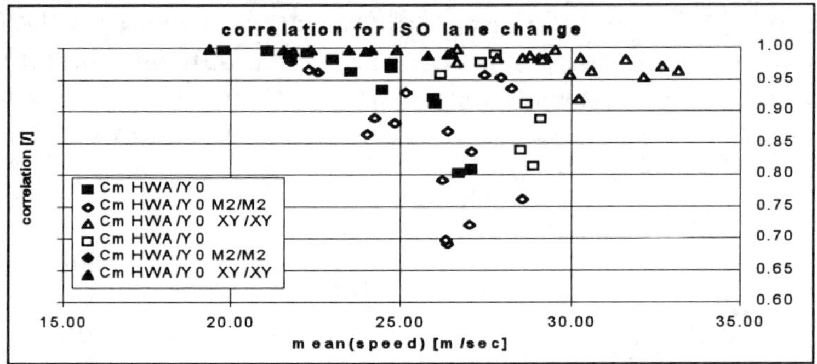

fig 16

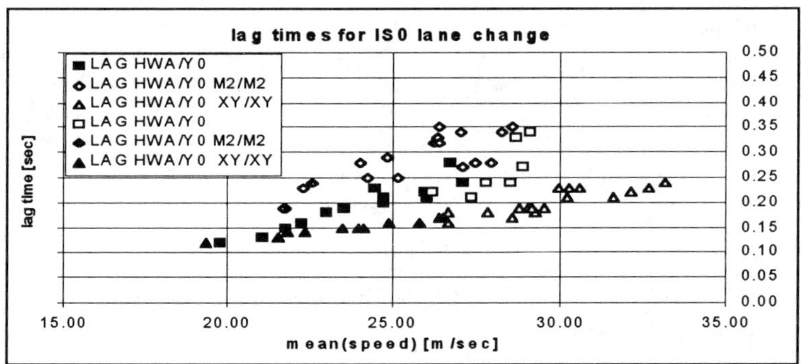

fig 17

indicated by squares, M2 tyres by diamonds and experimental tyres by triangles.

It is apparent that the experimental tyres have a marked performance advantage. They achieve the highest speed through the double lane change. However, the driver used a combination of steering and throttle control to achieve this goal. The limit speed established for constant throttle is similar to that achieved with standard tyres. The vehicle fitted with experimental tyres also maintained a very high correlation between the control input and corresponding vehicle response. The M2 tyres are inferior to the standard tyres, with the driver able to achieve speeds above 23 m/s only by using additional throttle control. Driver comments were consistent with the results discussed here. He reported that the experimental tyre fitment gave superior transient behaviour and grip.

Vehicle

Two modifications were carried out to the Jaguar test vehicle. Firstly a rack carrying 90 kg of ballast was fitted to its roof. The second chassis alteration involved the removal of the front anti-roll bar. Standard 225/55R16 Dunlop SP2000J tyres were fitted. Unfortunately, these tests were conducted in different seasons, and the results presented here may be influenced, to some extent, by changes in ambient temperature.

Results for peak correlation coefficients established for the hand wheel angle / lateral acceleration pair are illustrated in figure 18. Those concerning the vehicle for which the anti-roll bar is removed are denoted by diamonds, whereas triangles refer to the car fitted with the roof rack. Results of two failed tests obtained for each of the alternative set-ups are

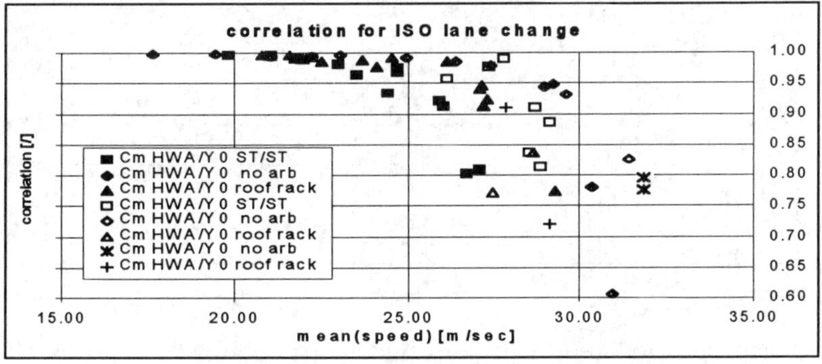

fig18

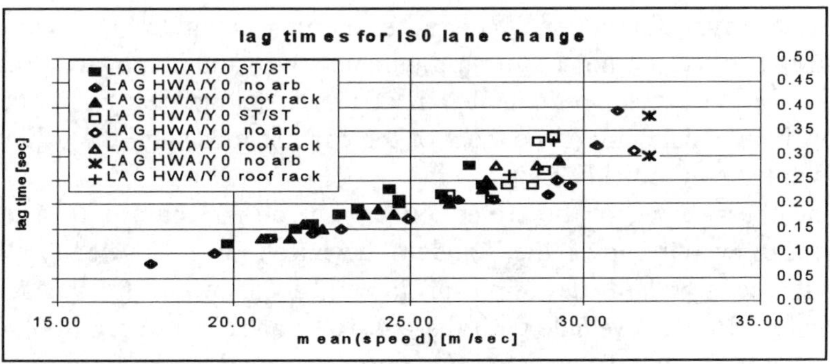

fig19

included. An asterisk (*) denotes failed tests for the car with its anti-roll bar removed. A cross (+) represents a failed test for a car equipped with the roof rack.

The onset of a decreasing lateral acceleration response occurs at a fairly high speed in the case of the vehicle with its anti-roll bar removed. The roof rack equipped Jaguar appears to have a sharper roll-off in behaviour compared to the progressively decreasing correlation coefficient obtained for the standard car. The lateral acceleration response of the former set-up remains well correlated to the steering input up to 27 m/s, before it deteriorates rapidly up to the limit speed of 29m/s.

Graphs indicating the time delays between steering and vehicle response show similar behaviour to that established for the corresponding cross correlation coefficients. Figure 19 shows those associated with lateral acceleration. The lateral response delays assume an almost constant rate of increase with manoeuvre severity. For the vehicle with its anti-roll bar removed, which features the lowest increase in delay at moderate

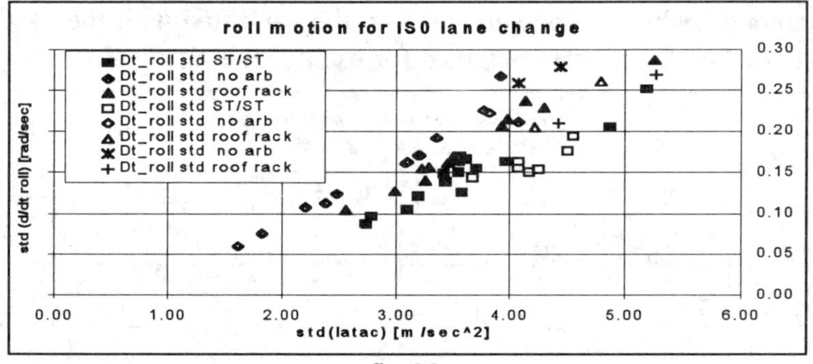

fig 20

speed, disproportionately high lag times were obtained at speeds close to the limit.

The test driver found this vehicle set-up unacceptable. He rejected it because it rolled too much during the manoeuvre, and commented that the vehicle felt 'unstable' on completion of the first lane change of the ISO Lane Change manoeuvre, the front of the car felt loose and the vehicle did not 'settle down' quickly enough.

The observations of the driver concerning roll motion are illustrated in figure 20, which shows the standard deviation of roll velocity plotted against the standard deviation of lateral acceleration (a measure of severity). Both the vehicle with the anti-roll bar removed and the vehicle with the roof rack fitted undergo more roll motion than the standard vehicle.

It is interesting to note that the vehicle with its anti-roll bar removed was rated as 'unacceptable', although it went through the lane change faster than possible with the other two set-ups. It appears that this test driver took more notice either, of the roll behaviour or the rate of change of the steering response near the limit, than of the vehicle's absolute performance.

10. CONCLUSIONS

Tyre property data, whether obtained by measurement or by using mathematical tyre models, can be used to derive tyre parameters which have been found to be broadly related to vehicle handling performance. However, the forces and moments generated by a tyre are sensitive to its vertical loading, and the angle which the tyre plane makes with the road surface. In a cornering manoeuvre, these factors are determined by the chassis characteristics of the vehicle to which the tyres are fitted. Mathematical models, which combine tyre and vehicle characteristics, provide a means of taking these factors into account and obtaining improved estimates of a tyre's handling properties on a specific vehicle. In addition, they enable vehicle handling like data to be obtained for development tyre designs, for which no physical prototype exists. Converting the model results into meaningful measures of handling quality is problematical. For the limit handling case, the use of cross correlation techniques appears to be a reasonable approach to this problem. There is some evidence that body roll itself, rather than its detrimental effect on a vehicle's lateral controllability, is a significant factor in the driver's perception of handling quality. More work is desirable in this area to investigate the appropriate weighting of these parameters.

REFERENCES

1. Pottinger, M. G., Marshall, K. D. and Arnold, G. A., 'Effect of Test Speed and Surface Curvature on Cornering Properties of Tires', *SAE paper No 760029.*
2. Barson, C. W., *Private Communication.*
3. Nordeen, D. L. 'Analysis of Tire Lateral Force and Interpretation of Experimental Tire Data', *Paper Presented at SAE National Meeting*, Jan 9-13 1967.
4. Pacejka, H, B, and Bakker E, 'The Magic Formula Tyre Model', *Tyre Models For Vehicle Dynamics Analysis, Supplement to Vehicle Systems Dynamics*, Vol. 21 pp1-18, 1993.
5. Hills, N., *Private Communication.*
6. Davies, V.E., *Private Communication.*
7. Jaksch, F.O., 'Driver Vehicle Interaction with Respect to Steering Controllability', *SAE paper No. 790740.*
8. Weir, D.H., DiMarco, R.J., 'Correlation and Evaluation of Driver/Vehicle Directional Response', *SAE paper No.780010.*
9. Sharp, R.S., *private communication.*

Vehicle Performance: J.P. Pauwelussen (ed.) pp. 196-217

Analysis of Ride Comfort Considering Driver Assessment

Detlef Kudritzki

1. INTRODUCTION

Optimization of ride comfort is gaining increasingly in importance in chassis development. Constantly rising traffic density and comfort-orientated customer preferences are mainly responsible for this. Comfort and its improvement are important, not only on bad road surfaces, but also on even surfaces. The cause is to be found in the increasing demand made on comfort [1,2,3,4]. It must also be considered that the expectations of the driver are of great importance. This means that on roads that, from the viewpoint of the driver, are good the driver obviously expects a lower vibration level. In spite of the importance of this factor and numerous studies on this field, a clear definition of ride comfort is lacking. On the one hand, the basic reason for this are the numerous investigations which would have to be carried out on the very different excitation profiles which the vehicle suspension system is subject to. The road surface is the input variable of the system. On the other hand, the output variables of the system to be evaluated are not sufficiently known [5,6]. This means that the correlation between the subjective assessment of ride comfort and the measurement of vehicle behavior is inadequately identified. The fundamental reason for this is that an exact definition of ride comfort, which is the basis is evaluating ride comfort, is lacking. This definition can be initially formulated in a descriptive way only. The description supplies the formulation for a measurement acquisition, as well as an evaluation of ride conditions which are confronted in making a subjective assessment [9,10,11].

It will be attempted to deliver a quantifiable measure of performance for assessing ride comfort where the preconceptions for a generally universal measurement description of ride comfort will not apply.
This means that the thresholds of the range of validity of assertions concerning ride comfort are reduced. These limitations refer to the input variables and output variables of the system vehicle, the drivers and the vehicles. The widely differing impressions which result, depending on the variation of the named parameters, make this step necessary. The mosaic-type connecting together of the individual results determined and partial correlations will yield a comprehensive description of ride comfort; that is hope for the future. In processing the results of ride comfort, identical methods of analysis are always employed.

2. DESCRIPTION OF RIDE COMFORT

A definition of ride comfort can be found only in the description of the interface between vehicle and driver. The interface consists of the contact points between driver and vehicle. These contact points are the sensory information channels of the human being. During the implementation of his driving task, the vehicle driver records the movements of the vehicle via his kinesthetic, acoustic and visual information channels.

The interface between driver and vehicle is the system output variable and provides the supply of information to the driver.
In the illustration the allocations of information channel to interface can be identified. The components consisting of seat, steering wheel, arm rests and floor form the interface both for the kinesthetic and for the tactile information channel. Both information channels record vibrations, using different sensors. From the point of view of ride comfort, the kinesthetic information channel is important, even if interference in the assessment of the vibration comfort through tactile-determined signals cannot be ruled out.

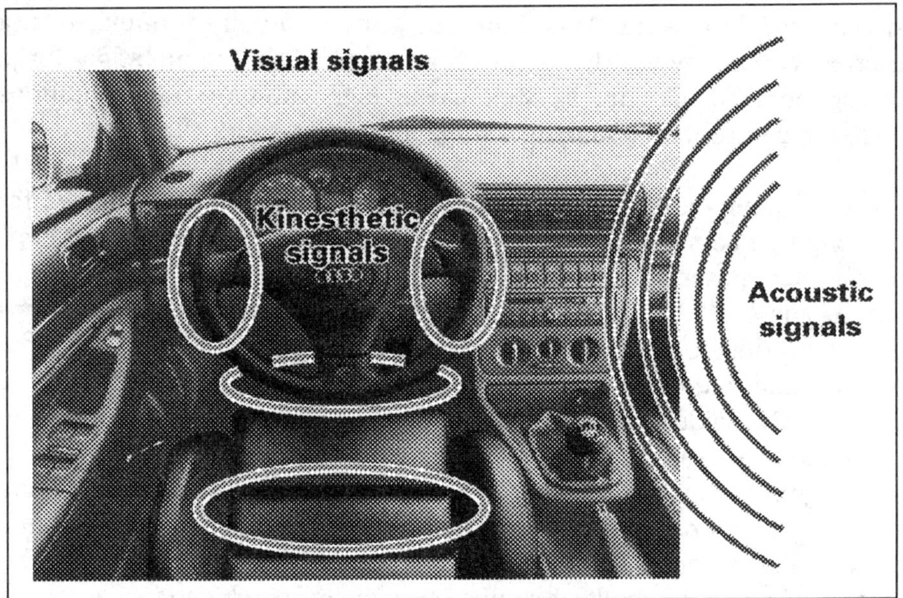

Fig. 1: Interface driver-vehicle

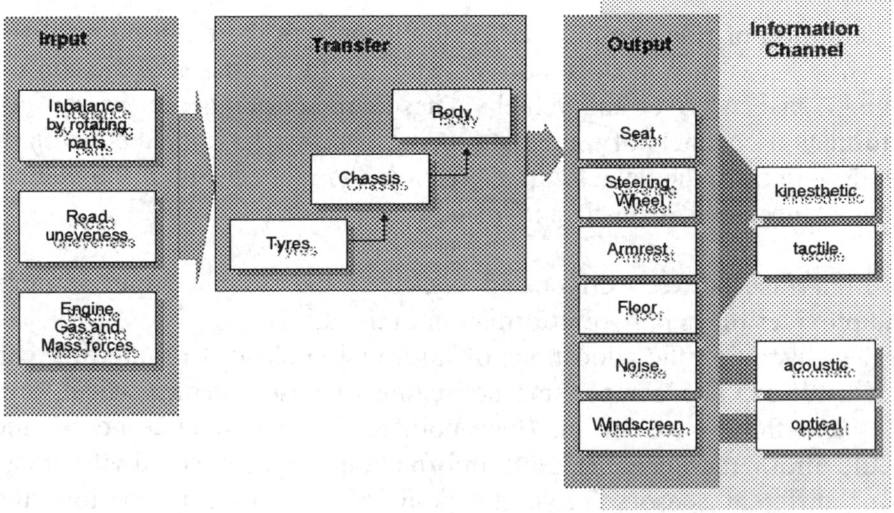

Fig. 2: Ride comfort-influencing parameters and their transfer path

The demand on vibrational behavior of the chassis means the following: No noise and no vibration in vehicle interior. Extensive studies have indicated that this principle is neither technically completely applicable, nor is it, with regard to the closed-cycle control system of driver-vehicle, necessary. The realistic demand on vibrational behavior, while considering the closed-cycle control system, therefore means: Insulation of vibrations which are perceived by the driver as unpleasant.

Ride comfort is achieved by optimized vibrational characteristic of chassis and car body. It is analyzed with the objective of studying vibrational behavior, where the frequency ranges (approx. 50 Hz) are relevant to the human body. The subjective perception of whole-body vibrations are most marked in the range 4 to 8 Hz [12].

Resonance frequency ranges for important parts of the body (vertical loading direction):

Head	20	[Hz]
Chest	10 - 50	[Hz]
Stomach	4 - 8	[Hz]
Pelvic area (2nd. Order)	10 - 12	[Hz]
Spine	10 - 12	[Hz]

The requirements of vibration-orientated design of the chassis can be referred to real driving situations. Excitations, which occur with small amplitude, should be capable of being absorbed so that they are not noticed by the driver. This is not possible for large displacement amplitudes. In the case of this type of excitation, the chassis is to be designed in such a way that the acceleration change for the vehicle occupant is reduced to a minimum, also in the case of intermittent stepwise excitation. The attenuation damping must be designed so that a resonant ringing of the chassis components in the vehicle interior is hardly audible. The vibration system to be considered consists of the following components: Tire, wheel, brake, spring, damper, steering wheel, bearing, subframe, power unit and car body (Fig. 3).

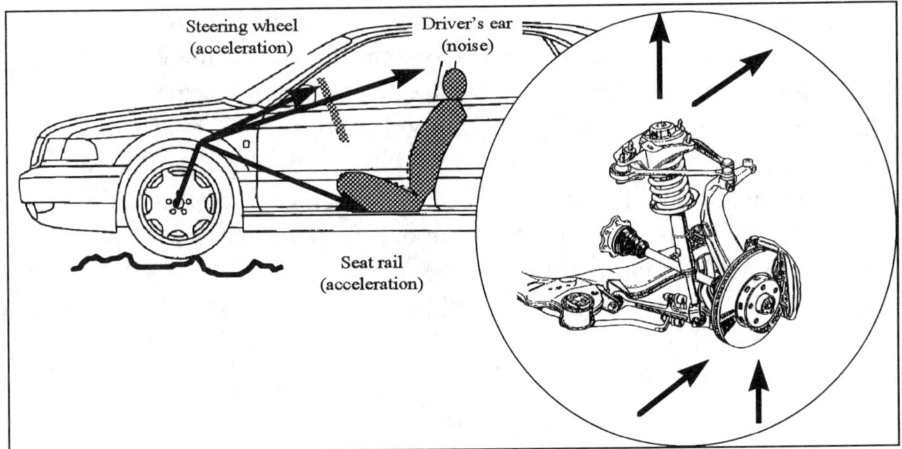

Fig. 3: Vibration transfer paths, caused by road surface

The system input variable is the road surface, while the system output variables are determined via the interface between driver and vehicle. For a better understanding of the movements occurring in the area of the wheel suspension, simpler models are initially employed (Fig. 4). Figure 4 likewise shows that a direct transform to the processes occurring during random driving surface stimulation is often not possible.

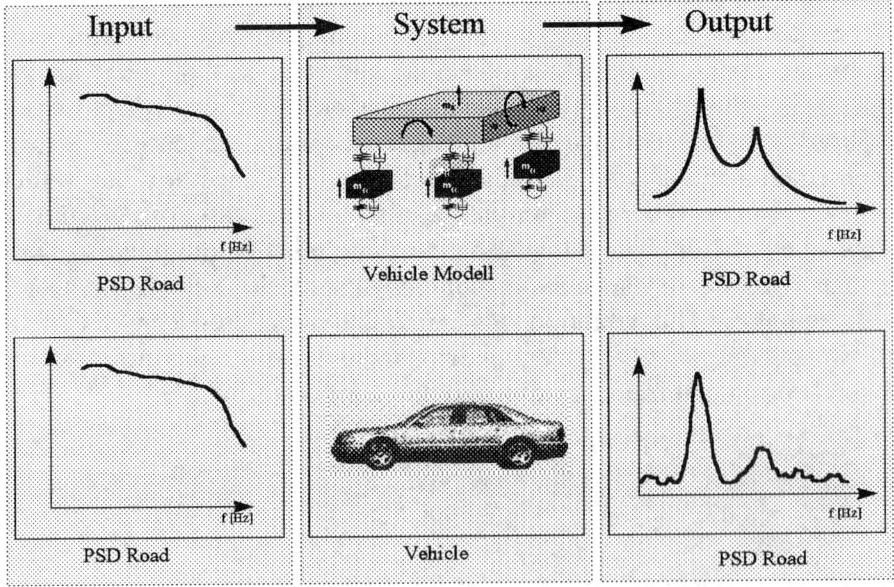

Fig. 4: Vehicle's NVH behavior

The demands made on the kinematics of the axles has resulted in structurally costly solutions, whose elastokinematics are no longer determined by the spring-damper strut alone. All linkages of the axles are connected with the car body via rubber-metal components. The vibration-orientated design of these components and that of the spring-damper strut is intimately related to the chassis stiffness properties. The vibration insulation of power unit and car body, using a subframe, places high demands on the power unit support, since, on the one hand, no chassis vibrations may be transmitted to the power unit and, on the other hand, power unit movement itself has to be insulated.

The demand on vibrational behavior of a modern chassis is a compromise between complete isolation of the road from the driver on the one hand and the transmission of necessary road information to the driver on the other.

3. ANALYSIS OF RIDE COMFORT

The analysis of ride comfort is based on a design development concept, which orientates itself to aspects of subjective vehicle assessment, objective technical-measurement description of the vehicle and simulation of vehicle behavior. In the following treatment driver assessment and vibration analysis are considered.

3.1 Design Development Concept

In order to carry out a structured analysis of ride comfort a predetermined concept of the fundamental procedure to be implemented is necessary. This essentially describes the development work necessary for the optimization of ride comfort. The necessary analyses for the study of vehicle behavior are carried out and adapted to one another against the background of this concept.

The objective of the analysis is the description and assessment of ride comfort. A forecast value must be found, which corresponds to the subjective judgment of the driver and which has been determined from parameters measured technically. For this, the correlations between the subjective assessment and the objective measuring data must be identified. The determined correlations must be confirmed through subjective assessment of ride comfort [13,14,15].

The methods of analysis presented in the following treatment can be assigned to 2 separate cycles, which are linked with each other and which form the development process. In the main cycle, the correlation between subjective assessment and objective measured values is determined. The chassis is optimized in the secondary cycle with respect to this. The secondary cycle is the developmental cycle where an assessment and analysis of ride comfort, based on the knowledge of the correlation between objective and subjective data, are carried out. Mutual dependencies exist between both cycles,.

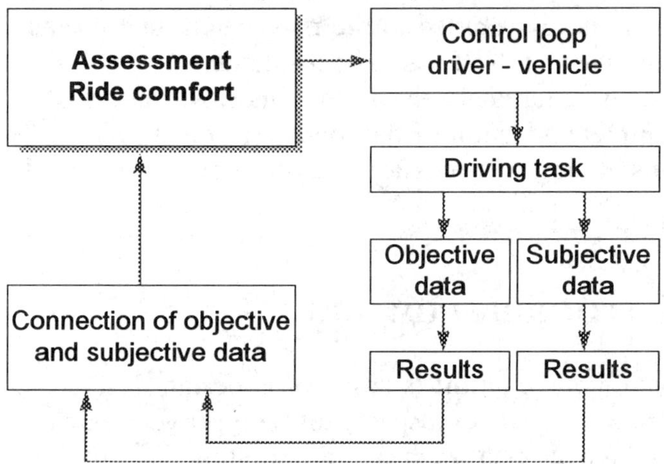

Fig. 5 : Assessment cycle: Correlation of subjective and objective data

In the assessment cycle, the closed-cycle control system must be defined first. Driver and vehicle characteristics are to be defined and selected in a manner which is adapted to the object of investigation. The interface driver-vehicle determines the measurement points. In the case of the driving task it must be considered that the subject of assessment is perceptible. The experiments should be carried out blind. The objective data is the measuring data, processed in the form of characteristic values. The subjective data is derived from the assessments of the drivers [16]. They should be implemented in relation to a reference vehicle. The prepared data groups are correlated by means of a linking method.

The development cycle of chassis optimization describes a part of the main cycle. It documents the ride test, including the analysis and the assessment. The measured variables are to be selected in such a way that they describe both system behaviour for vehicle and the interface between driver and vehicle. In parallel with the measurement data, the subjective ride impression is gained. The interpretation of the measurement data, taking into consideration the subjective assessment, defines an optimized component, which activates a new development cycle when integrated into the vehicle.

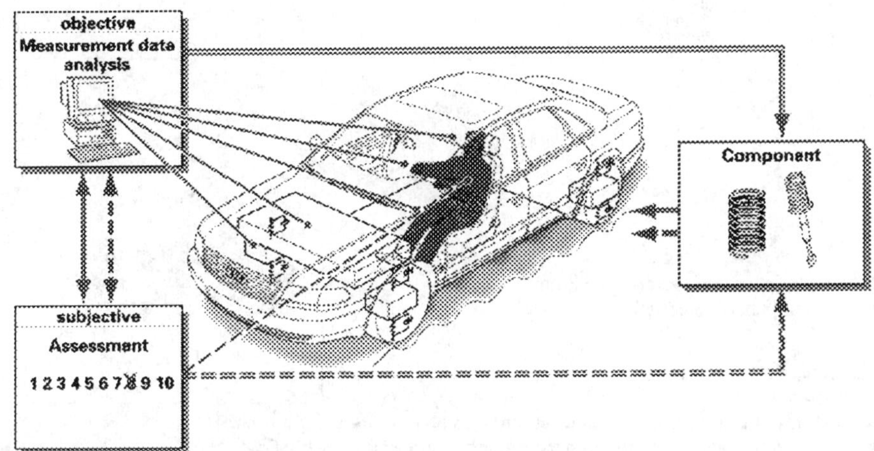

Fig. 6: Chassis optimization development cycle

3.2 Methods Of Analysis

The methods of analysis are subdivided within the design development concept. In these methods, all processes, which are the leading indicators (according to state-of-the-art know-how) in achieving correct interpretation of comfort-related vibrational behavior, are integrated.

The methods of analysis used are dependent on the operation steps to be implemented in the entire development process.

The multiple correlation is applied as a method of forming a link between objective and subjective data, for processing objects of investigation in the processing cycle. By means of multiple correlation, an equation for predicting a criterion variable (subjective judgment) is determined on the basis of several predictor variables (objective characteristic values). A linear extension (regression), based on experience gained, leads to a sufficiently good result quality.

In the design development cycle, a large number of analysis procedures are available [17,18]. Basically the following is valid: Only processes, which are capable of being securely controlled and where the interpretation potentialities are known, are utilized.

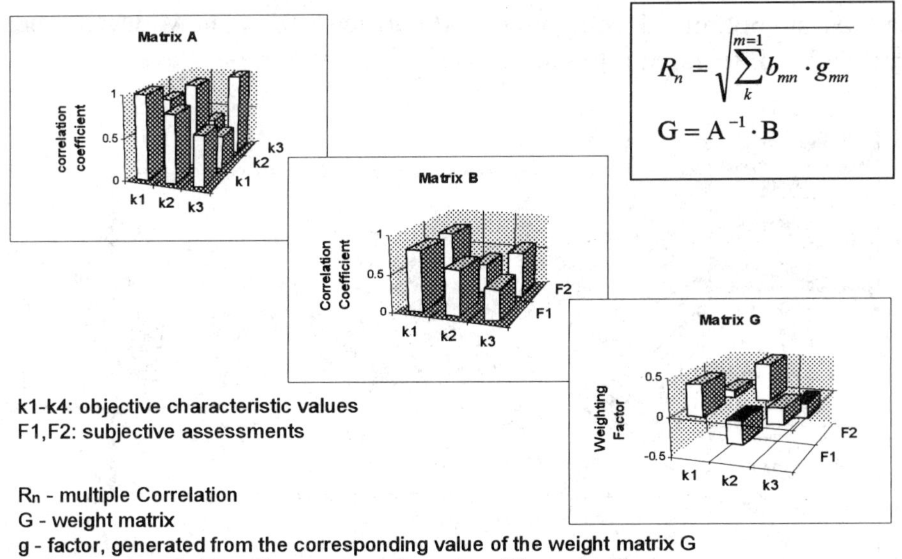

$$R_n = \sqrt{\sum_k^{m=1} b_{mn} \cdot g_{mn}}$$

$$G = A^{-1} \cdot B$$

k1-k4: objective characteristic values
F1,F2: subjective assessments

R_n - multiple Correlation
G - weight matrix
g - factor, generated from the corresponding value of the weight matrix G
b - factor, generated from the corresponding value of the matrix B
A - matrix from the individual correlation of the objective data
B - matrix from individual correlations fromobjective and subjective dates

Fig. 7: Intermediate steps for determining the multiple correlation

The selection of a suitable analysis procedure depends both on the point of time within the design development cycle and also depends on complexity of the system to be investigated. In the case of system concepts the overall system is considered fundamentally, resulting from this the system is then broken down into sub-systems. The checking of development steps is implemented over the entire system as a whole.
A typical design development cycle begins with the subjective assessment of the actual status. Based on these ride tests, a measurement is made of the total vehicle. The test route and the test setup depend on the subjective assessment ride. The evaluations in the time and frequency range are a result of the problem description and the task definition. Based on the measurements carried out on the total vehicle, the vibration system which is relevant for optimization, can be designated. This leads to a definition of the operating vibration analysis, that is itself connected into the design development cycles. It is used for visualization purposes and for the identification of weak points. Detailed questions relating to specific components are processed using modal analysis. A more detailed description of the vibration system is then implemented on the hydropulse system. Concurrent considerations of the vibration system on the vehicle model assist understanding and parameter variation. The subsequent component optimization is carried out on the function test

stand. The application of the thus redefined component concludes the development cycle and is simultaneously the starting point for the next cycle.

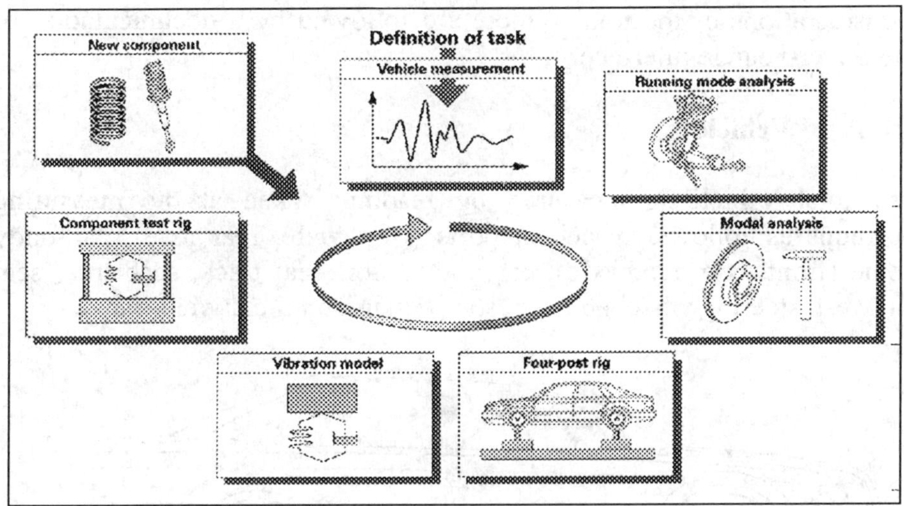

Fig. 8: Working tools in the development cycle

The tests to be carried out within the framework of vibration analysis are fundamentally decided as a result of the ride tests and stand tests. In both cases, total vehicle and vehicle components are stimulated with deterministic and non-deterministic signals.

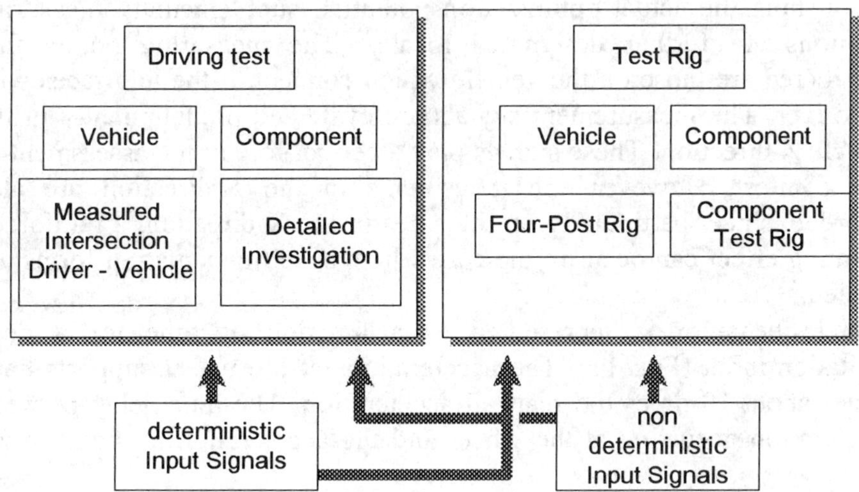

Fig. 9: Test conditions

4. RESULTS

The results determined from the analysis methods are presented in the following text. The main focus is on the presentation of basic findings. Considerations of the total vehicle are followed by a documentation of the driver-vehicle interface.

4.1 Total Vehicle

The total vehicle is measured by readings taken at the measuring positions as follows; wheel supports (front axle, rear axle), car body dome (front axle, rear axle), car body floor, seat track, seat area, seat backrest, steering wheel and acoustic pressure on the driver's ear.

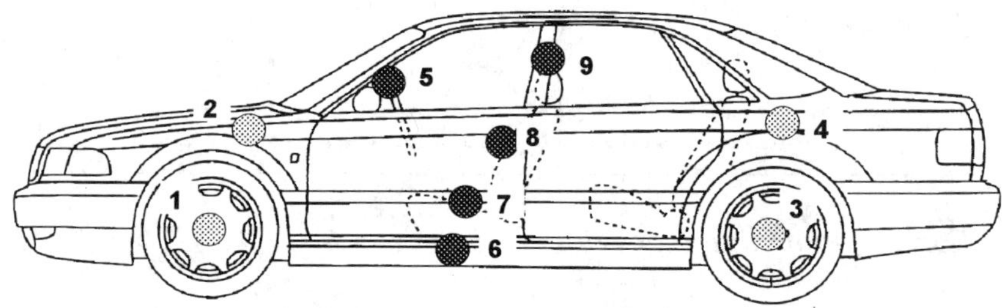

Fig. 10: Measuring points for documentation of the total vehicle

These measuring points are used if the actual status condition is documented at the beginning of the analysis. In the process of establishing the actual optimization potential, supplementary measuring positions are further designated locally. The measuring points first considered are those on the vehicle which connect to the interfaces with the driver. The measurement signals are evaluated predominantly in the vehicle Z-direction. These signals play a central role in the assessment of ride comfort. However, the movements in the X-direction are also recorded, since, particularly on the axles in the X-direction, a reinforced vibrating effect can occur in the case where specific excitation forms are applied.

Vehicle behavior is represented as a function of time for a peak excitation input (Fig. 11). The accelerations at the wheel supports have values about 10 times the seat rail acceleration. The time delay between acceleration occurring at the wheel and the acceleration at the seat can also be identified clearly. The difference in period of the measurement signals at the different positions is also striking.

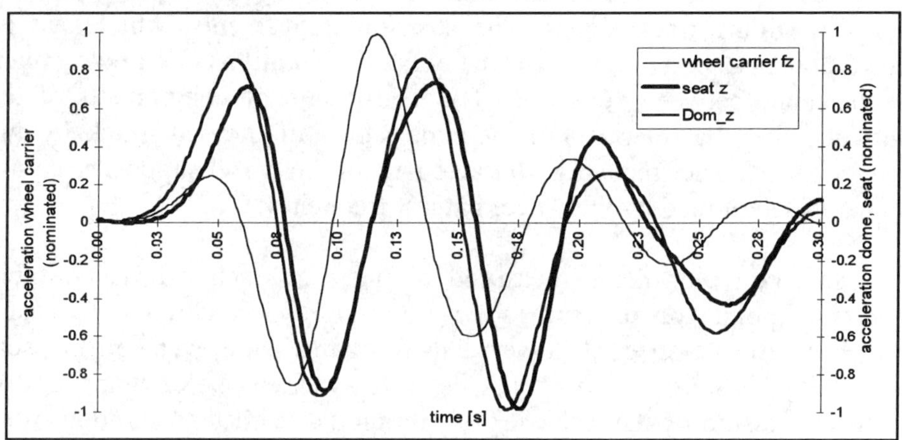

Fig. 11: Time history of accelerations caused by peak input at front axle

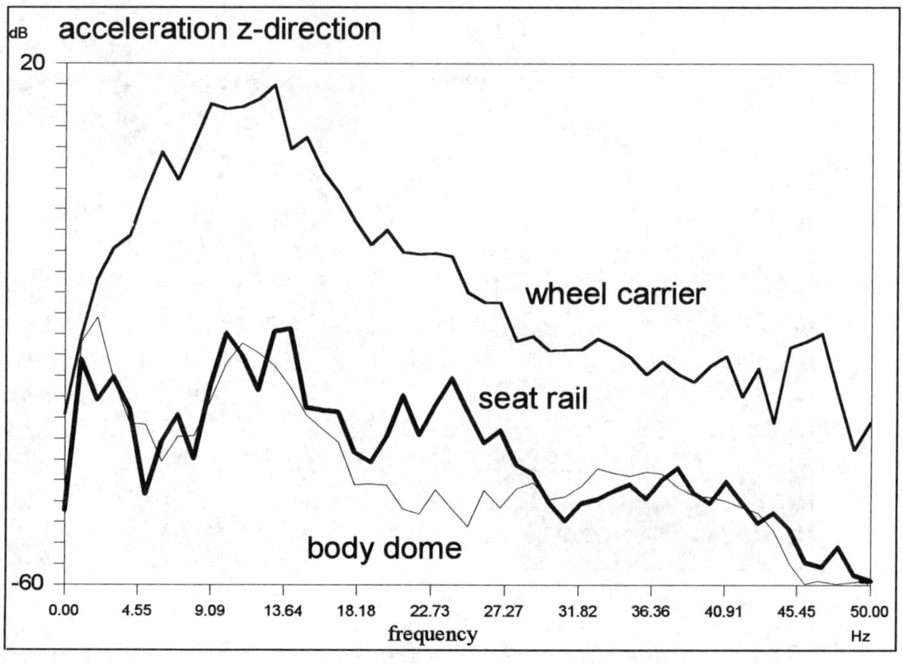

Fig. 12: Spectral power density at the wheel support structure, dome and seat track

208   D. KUDRITZKI

The frequency components of the time plots histories illustrated in Fig.
11 are outlined in Fig. 12. It is obvious that some frequency components,
which are not identified at the wheel supports, are contained clearly in
the seat sliding track signal. The structure movements, which can be
noted at the car body dome, and the car body vibrations, are predominant
in the range between 20 and 30 Hz. The frequency components of the
structure are characterized in the time signal of the seat track by the
longer period. The frequency characteristic of the wheel support structure
signal is determined by the wheel natural frequency.

The spectral color maps measured at the seat track offer a suitable
reference point for the subjective ride impression (Fig. 13). Taken
together with the spectral power density of the same event on the seat
track (Fig. 14), ride comfort can be well assessed. Color maps give a
good impression of the intensity of vibrations. With discontinuous step
excitation (Fig. 13), the decay of the vibrations can also be evaluated.

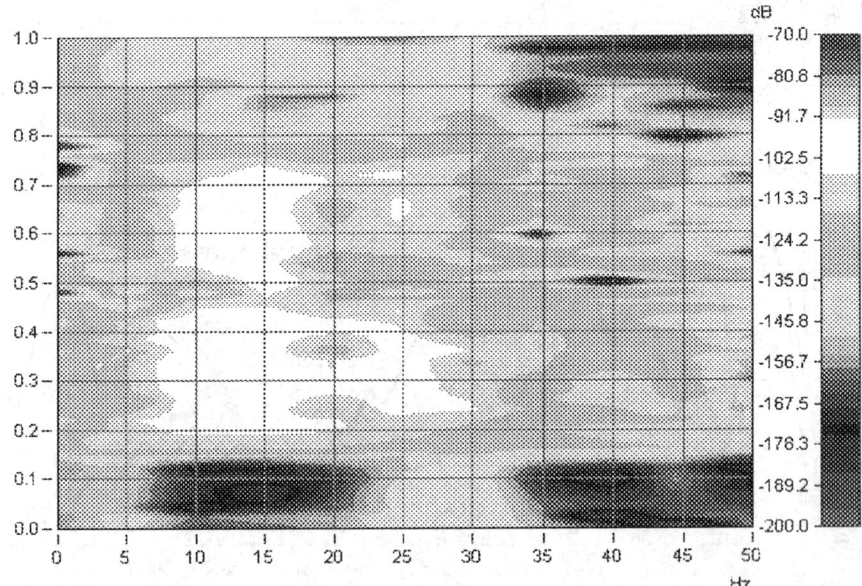

*Fig. 13: Spectral color map of the seat track acceleration, caused by an
input step*

Driving over an input step can be recognized clearly in Fig. 13, first with
the front axle and then with the rear axle. In the color map, bright areas
indicate high vibration level. The importance of the traveling speed can

be recognized in this illustration. According to this illustration, if the traveling speed is increased, the vibrations of front and rear axle overlap. On the other hand, the velocity must be selected in such a way that the physical effects to be examined occur in actual practice. It is known that car body vibrations are permanently present, while vibrations in the range of the wheel natural frequency only occur in the case of more severe driving surface stimuli: In these cases, however, with higher levels.

A more detailed analysis of the vibrations occurring is possible, as shown in the representation of the frequency range in Fig. 14. A suitable selection of excitation form, sampling rate, filter and time window means that the vibration characteristic behavior of a vehicle can be well identified. The peaks that occur can be assigned to specific components. By means of well-defined allocation, the objective of optimization of the individual components can also be achieved. Nevertheless, the measures applied for the purposes of vibration optimization must be tuned to each other.

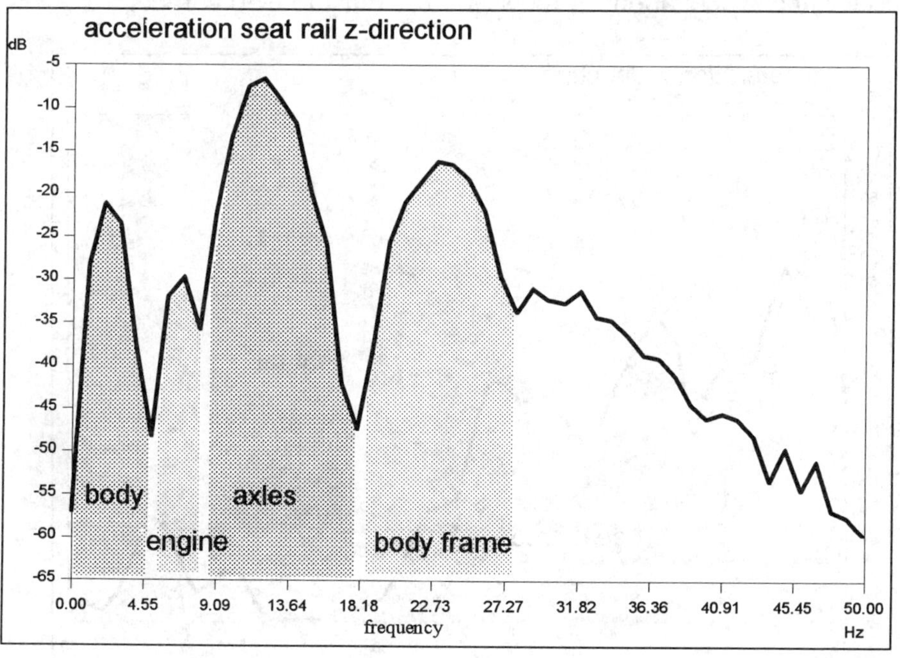

Fig. 14: Spectral power density (same event as Fig. 13)

4.2 Seating

Seating comfort is described by the following factors:

- Vibration behavior
- Ergonomics
- Seating comfort
- Seat pressure distribution
- Orthopedic considerations

For the study of ride comfort, vibration behavior of the above items is of exceptional importance. The accelerations are measured on the seat track, seat area and seat backrest in 3 directions. Seat pressure distribution is especially important in considering the lay-out and the positioning of the seat sensors.

Measurements on the seat on uneven road surfaces are detailed in Fig. 15. Illustrated are the spectral power densities of the seat track and seat cushion in the Z-direction. In order to represent the driver-vehicle interface, the accelerations at the seat areas must to be recorded.

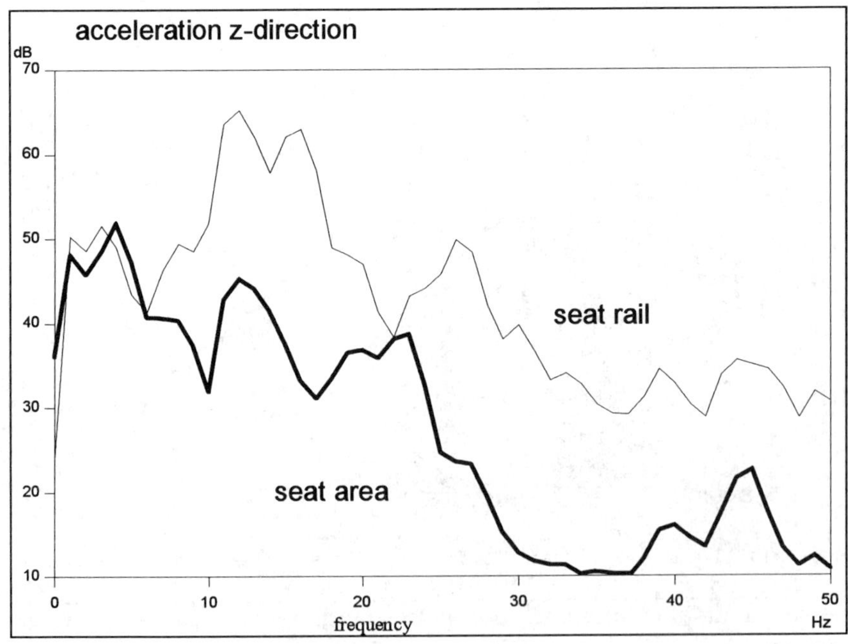

Fig. 15: Spectral power density of the seat for uneven road surface

On the other hand, it must be considered that the signals on the seat track disperse to a lesser degree and seating comfort is influenced by the use of a sensor in the seat. As a result of comprehensive studies it was found that the acceleration on the seat track turned out be a meaningful parameter variable in assessing ride comfort. However, in the lay-out of the seating and basic investigative studies on subject of ride comfort, the recording of vibrations at the seat area cannot be dispensed with. In figure 15, the vibration-impeding action of the seat can be seen. For the assessment of ride comfort, the frequency range is considered up to 30 [Hz]. Fig. 16 shows the corresponding transfer function with typical increase in the range of approx. 5 [Hz].

The problems involved in the installation of a seat sensor are clearly illustrated in Fig. 17. The thin line shows the spectral power density when the sensor is located in the range of the coccyx. It is called the normal position because it is in this area that the highest seat pressure occurs. If the sensor is in the front area of the seat, the measurement result is falsified.

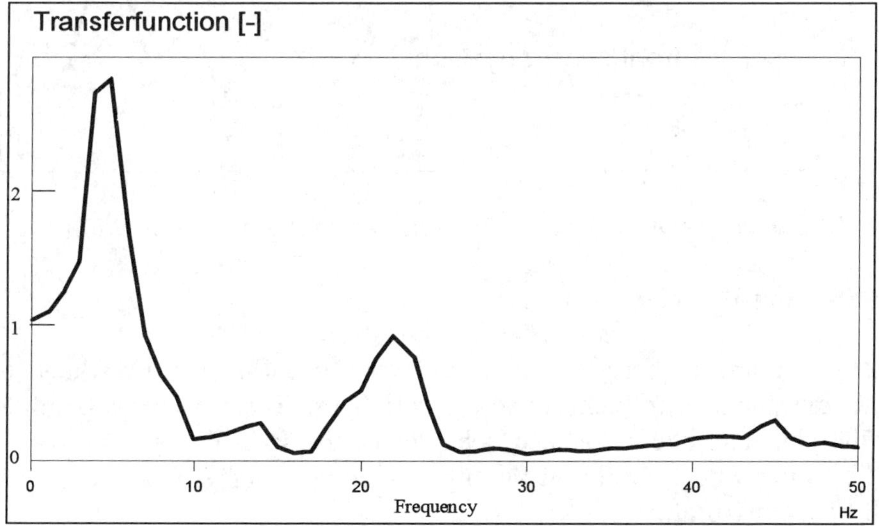

Fig. 16: Transfer function seat area/seat rail

It causes a displacement of the peaks and a more severe attenuation damping in the frequency range above 30 [Hz]. Vibration behavior of a seat can be assessed exactly by the driver. Apparently the frequency range up to 30 [Hz] is the range which the driver the driver is aware of.

The resonant frequency of the seat was of subordinate importance, since no higher levels occur in this range in the frequency spectrum (Fig. 15). In any case the resonant frequency of the seat may not lie in the range of resonance of other vehicle components (e.g. engine).

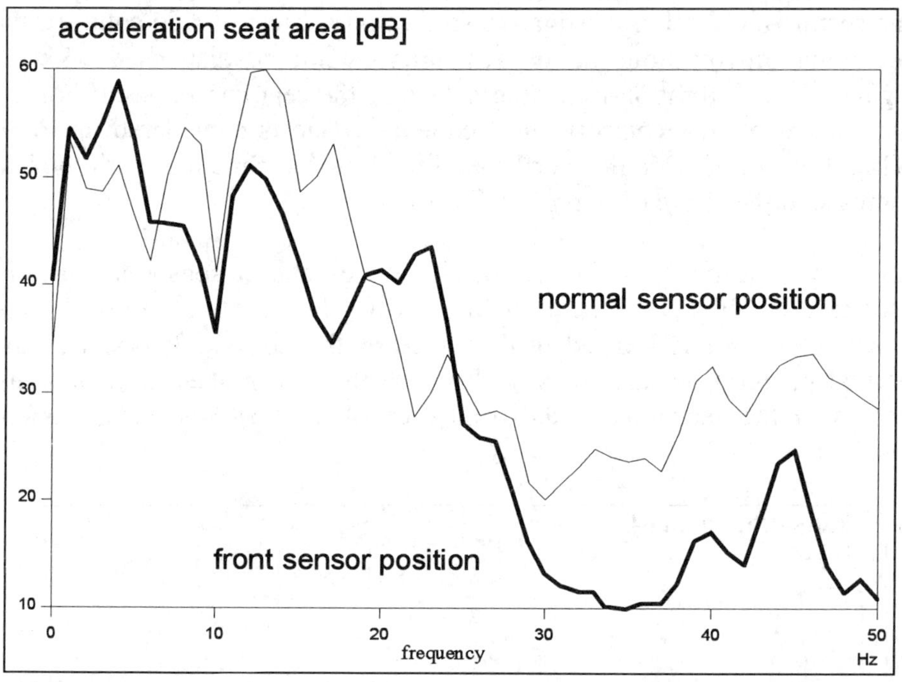

Fig. 17: Spectral power density, influenced by the sensor's position

4.3 Steering Wheel

A further interface between driver and vehicle is the steering wheel. Its vibrations can also influence ride comfort. The vibrations are determined by the characteristic resonance behavior of the steering column system and steering wheel, while on the other hand steering gear and car body will transmit vibrations.

In Fig. 18, the influence caused by the intensity of the grip on the steering wheel is documented. What is striking is the severe increase in vibrations in the range 25-30 [Hz], when the steering wheel is released. The forearm indicates a resonance frequency range from 15-30 [Hz] so that these vibrations of the steering column are still in a sensitive range. A shaking and a prickling feeling in the steering wheel to 150 [Hz] can be noticeably perceived.

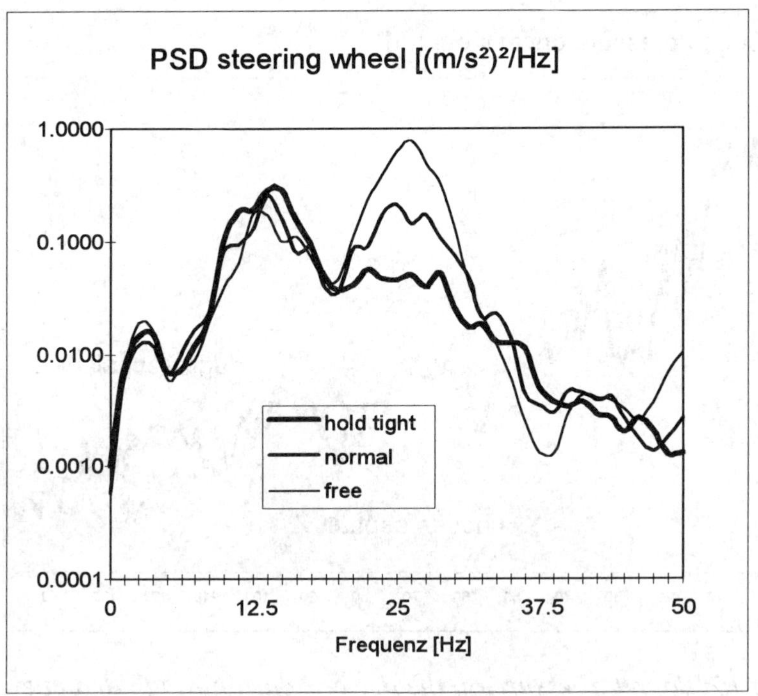

Figure 18: Influence on the measurement result of the intensity of grip on the steering wheel

4.4 Acoustic Pressure

The acoustic pressure is the acoustic interface of the driver to the vehicle. The acoustic comfort impression is strongly formed by the acoustic pattern. For this reason, in the case of detailed acoustic study, the entire frequency range of audible vibrations must be recorded. In this treatment, the frequency range, which has a direct connection to low-frequency vibrations described already, is considered. Fig. 19 shows the different effect impressions of the acoustic pressure while driving over uneven and rough asphalt. The high-frequency portions of the rough asphalt can be clearly identified.

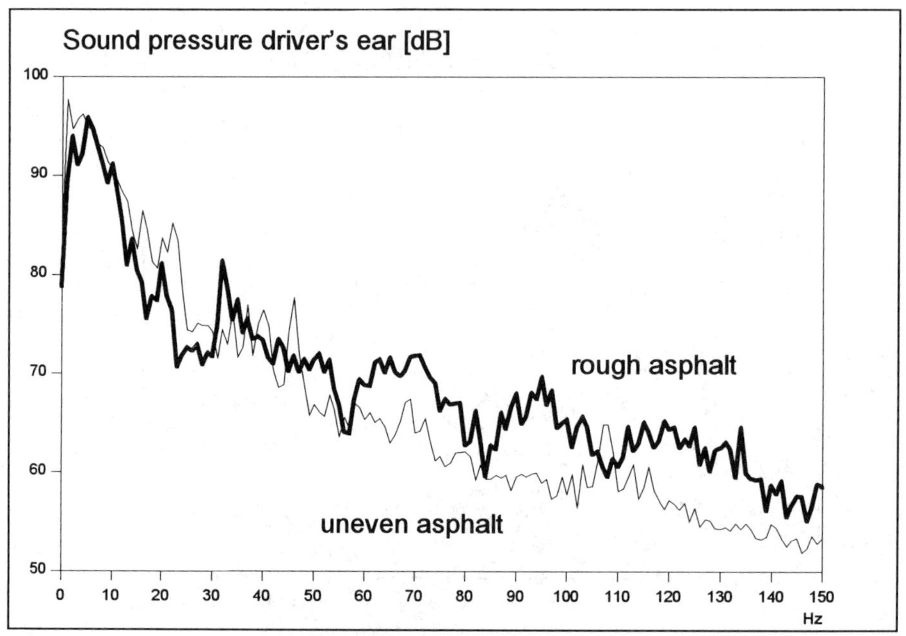

Figure 19: Sound pressure on the driver's ear on rough and uneven asphalt

5. CONCLUSIONS

The ride comfort of a vehicle can be described using the driver-vehicle interface by measurement of the acceleration applied to the seat and steering wheel, as well as the acoustic pressure on the driver's ear. The vibration behavior of the interface is documented for deterministic and non-deterministic excitations. The vibration analysis of the system is implemented using synthetic excitations, while the subjective ride impression on natural highways is recorded and interpreted verbally and with measurements.

An assessment and analysis of ride comfort, with a good approximation to subjective evaluation, can be carried out in compressed form by means of the seat track rail signal.

Since no comprehensive assessment is possible with this variable, a tabular representation of the relevant sizes is provided for summary purposes:

Acceleration of seat track rail   Z-direction   to 30 [Hz]
Acceleration of steering wheel   Z-direction   to 40 [Hz]
Acoustic pressure on the driver's ear   to 150 [Hz]

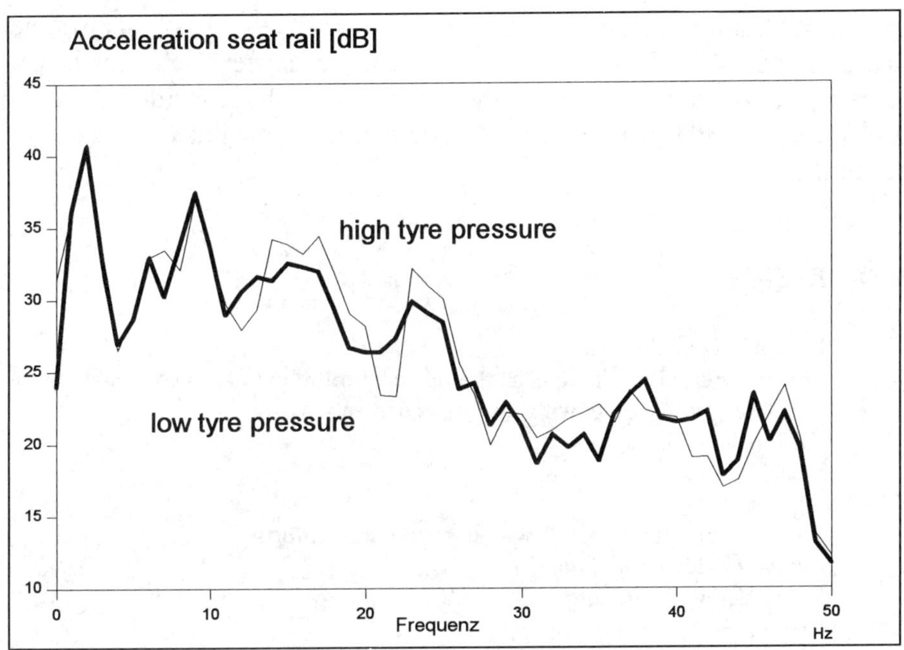

igure 20: Influence of tire inflation pressure on acceleration of the seat track rail

Fig. 20 shows the spectral power densities of the seat track rail while driving over a step input. The tire pressure was selected in the example as a comfort-influencing parameter, in order to cause a modification of ride comfort for all driver-vehicle interfaces. The tire pressure was varied in such a way that the influence on ride comfort could be perceived subjectively. The level in the range of the wheel natural frequency and of the car body vibrations could be lowered by about 2-3 [dB], by a reduction of the tire pressure. The partial interface formed by the seat is documented in part in representation Fig. 20. Behavior occurring as a result of other excitations must also be considered. Since it is a question of transient processes, the time characteristic plot of vibrations must be considered as well.

The aim of the analysis of ride comfort is the optimization of vibration characteristic behavior. For this purpose the connection between measurement parameters and the subjective assessment of ride comfort must be analyzed even more intensively. Detailed consideration of the total vehicle with all interfaces is necessary at first, then partial interfaces must also be studied in detail. The studies are to be carried out by specialists and customers. Since the analyses have component optimization as the final aim, a consideration of system behavior is vital. Here not only is the system output variable to be considered i.e. the driver-vehicle interface, but also the transfer path must also be taken into account.

REFERENCES

/1/   Pelargus, D.; Schmidt, A.
The influence of oscillations on the ride comfort of passenger cars: a study to correlate objective data with subjective perceptions
SAE paper 925183
FISITA 1992

/2/   Rericha, I.
Methoden zur objektiven Bewertung des Fahrkomforts
Automobil-Industrie 2/86, S.175-182
Vogel-Verlag, Würzburg

/3/   Parsons, K.C.; Griffin, M.J.
Methods for predicting passenger vibration discomfort
SAE Technical Series, SAE-831029, 1983

/4/   Hennecke, D.
Zur Bewertung das Schwingungskomforts von Pkw bei instationären Anregungen
VDI Fortschritt-Berichte Nr. 237
VDI-Verlag Düsseldorf, 1994

/5/   Takata,N.; Ikura,S.; Shimada, T.
A consideration on analysis of ride harshness
JSAE review, Tokyo, 13.3.1984, S. 54-59

/6/   Norsworthy, T. H.
The correlation of objective ride measures to subjective jury evaluations of class 8 coe vehicles
SAE paper 850985

/7/   Kozawa, Y.; Sugimoto, G.; Suzuki, Y.
A new ride comfort meter
SAE paper 860430
Int. Congress, Detroit, Mi, 1986

/8/   Laermann, F.-J.; Koenigsfeld, H.
Verbesserungen von Komfort und Fahrverhalten durch adaptive Änderung von Fahrwerksparametern
SAE paper 865113, 1986

/9/   Simic, D.
Beitrag zur Optimierung der Schwingungseigenschaften des Fahrzeuges: Physiologische Grundlagen des Schwingungskomforts
Dissertation, TU Berlin, 1970

/10/   Cucuz, S.

Schwingempfinden von Pkw-Insassen, Auswirkungen von stochastischen Unebenheiten und Einzelhindernissen der realen Fahrbahn
Dissertation, TU Braunschweig, 1992

/11/   Buck, B.; Knoblauch, J.; Wölfel, H.
Ein Schwingungsdummy zur objektiven und reproduzierbaren Messung der Schwingungseinwirkung auf den sitzenden Menschen.
VDI-Berichte Nr. 1189, 1995, S.275-284

/12/   Brüel & Kjær
Humanschwingungen
Info-Broschüre, 1. issue 10/89

/13/   Sano, S.; Furukawa, Y; Oguchi, Y; Nakaya, H.
Effects of Vehicle Response Characteristics and Driver's Skill Level on Task Performance and Subjective Rating

/14/   DIN 45 676
Mechanical driving-point impedance and transmissibility of the human body
Deutsche Norm 11/92

/15/   Salvendy, G.
Handbook of Human Factors
John Wiley & Sons 1987; S. 48,49

/16/   Rohrmann, B.
Empirische Studien zur Entwicklung von Antwortskalen für die sozialwissenschaftliche Forschung
Zeitschrift für Sozialpsychologie 1978, 9, S.222-245

/17/   Bukovics, J.; Rau, R.; Young, D. J.
Fahrkomfort: Mess-und Analyseverfahren als Hilfsmittel bei der Fahrzeugentwicklung
VDI-Bericht Nr. 791
Tagung Mess-und Versuchstechnik im Automobilbau, München 1990

/18/   Hieronimus, K.
Zum Einsatz von Berechnungs- und Versuchstechniken bei der schwingungstechnischen und akustischen Entwicklung von Pkw
Tagung Meß- und Versuchstechnik im Automobilbau, München 4/1990
VDI Berichte 791

Vehicle Performance: J.P. Pauwelussen (ed.) pp. 218-229

Vehicle Occupant Response to Noise - Psycho-acoustic Concepts and Analysis Methods

D.G.Fish

1. OVERVIEW

The issue of correlating occupant response to vehicle interior noise with objective parameters is a subject that has preoccupied automotive engineers for some time, and will continue to do so for many years to come. Although the ideal of perfect correlation of subjective and objective data is unlikely to be achieved, the techniques used to highlight subject response can have a significant effect on improving the information and correlation gained. At the centre of this lies the individual subject inconsistencies in response, and the disagreements between subjects. Both phenomena are prevalent in the automotive world, and cannot be disregarded when investigating such issues.

The approach considered here covers the use of the pair-comparison technique and multidimensional scaling to understand and overcome these issues. A worked example has been used to illustrate the problem; that of power-steering noise which occurs during low speed turning manoeuvres.

1. THE CASE HISTORY

Power-steering noise represents a typical acoustic phenomenon that occurs in most modern cars. The source of excitation is such that the frequencies observed by the driver are directly a function of the rotation speed of the pump, and the number of pulses generated within the system (figure 1). In this case the key harmonic components are 10, 20,, and 30 times rotation speed of the pump. In the vehicle these are combined with other vehicle noise sources such as engine, road and wind noise which act as a form of masking. Through engineering investigation of pump designs, significant changes in the 'character' of pump noise observed inside the vehicle can be achieved. In objective terms these are observed through both amplitude and phase effects. In addition, changes in the background noise level have also been found to affect the perception of the power-steering pump noise. Clearly there are a number of issues here which can be influenced by pump design, and have varying influence upon the subject response. However, because of the mechanisms associated with power-steering pump noise it is not always possible to make changes that affect only one of the pump characteristics at anyone time. To understand the individual subjective significance of each component in the noise it is necessary to breakdown the subject response. Traditional rating schemes cannot satisfactorily achieve this since two sounds can have the same overall rating yet be totally different in character. To this end the pair comparison technique was used and implemented as described below.

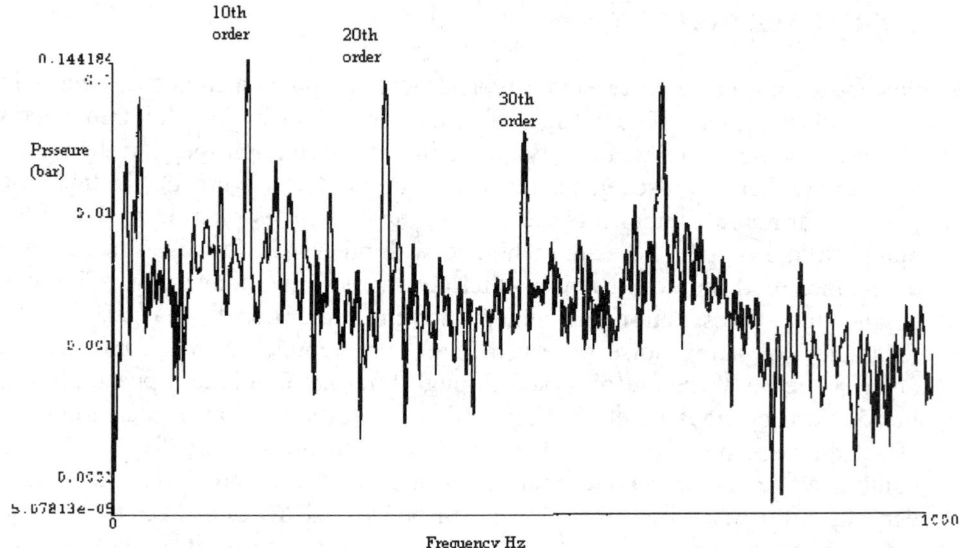

Figure 1 Typical harmonic content from a power-steering pump

3. EXPERIMENTAL ISSUES

3.1 Rating Scales versus Pair Comparison

Rating scales and pair comparisons are two methods used for subjectively assessing vehicle noise.

The rating scheme used at MIRA is as follows:

Rating

1 - No operation
2 - Limited operation
3 - Complained as bad failure by all occupants
4 - Rated as failure by all occupants
5 - Rated as disturbing by all occupants
6 - Rated disturbing by some occupants
7 - Noticeable by all occupants
8 - Noticeable by only critical occupants
9 - Noticeable only to trained evaluators
10 - Not noticeable to trained evaluators

The pair comparison technique is well established as a method of comparing a number of sounds. The detail of the technique can be found in reference 1. It's advantage over the rating scale method can be summarised below:

- yields more information
- allows detailed analysis
- allows application of multi-dimensional scaling
- more robust for naïve subjects
- no drift in opinion

The main disadvantages of the pair comparison technique are:

- time consuming
- tedious for the subject
- yields only relative data
- can only be applied in laboratory, and not with real vehicle evaluation

Clearly therefore there are a number of limitations with the pair comparison technique. However, the information that it can yield can lead to a better understanding of rating scale evaluations of the same sounds, and therefore ultimately assist in developing a subjective tool for the prediction of occupant response to the noise.

3.2 Subject inconsistencies (coefficient of consistency)

The analysis techniques for subject responses are important not only for establishing basic facts about the validity of the subject response data gathered, but it can also provide important information upon the spread of subject responses. Analysis of subject categories can help establish whether bi-variance in the subject responses is in evidence or not, whereas information on individual responses and agreement between subjects can throw light on the general population spread. Knowledge of the nature of the data is important in helping to decide which types of correlation analysis are applicable to the data, and also gives an indication as to the limitations of statistical techniques applied.

Consider the following scenario. A subject is asked to judge his or her preference for three noises A, B, and C. Let the fact that A is preferred to B be denoted by the notation A $\longrightarrow$ B, or B $\longleftarrow$ A, in other words the direction of the arrow indicates the direction of decreasing preference. If the subject responds with

A ⟶ B and B ⟶ C, then we would logically expect the subject to select A⟶ C. If, however, the subject chose C ⟶ A instead of A ⟶ C, then the overall response would be inconsistent; a likely scenario. For more than three stimuli there is obviously more than one potential circular triad. The Coefficient of Consistency (K) is a linear function of the number of circular triads in evidence in an individuals complete response. It returns a value of one for complete consistency, and a value of zero for total inconsistency. Figure 2 illustrates two levels of consistency that can typically occur. In the first case there are no inconsistent triads, whereas in the second case all possible triads are inconsistent.

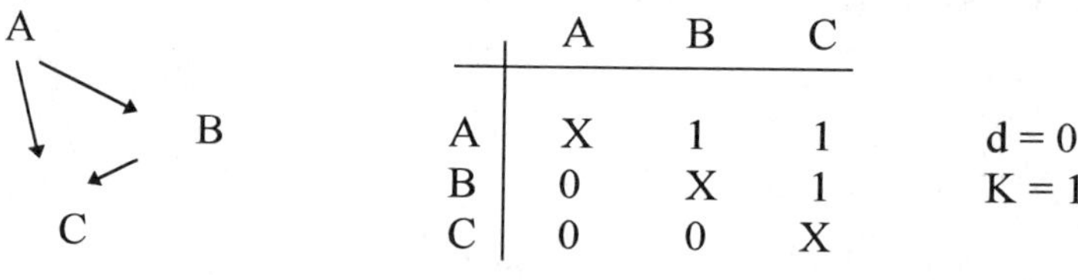

Figure 2 Consistent and inconsistent responses

d - Number of incomplete triads
K - Coefficient of consistency

In general, experience has shown that subjects become more inconsistent for less variance in dBA between stimuli. This is not a surprising observation. There are a number of possible explanations for inconsistency in subjective response:

a)   The subject is not concentrating at all in the experiment and is making random or uninformed choices.

b)   The subject is unable to decide between stimuli in terms of preference, and so their choice becomes arbitrary.

c)   The subjects perception of noise changes with time.

d)   The subjects are using different criteria in their assessment of pairs of stimuli within the same group.

Clearly these explanations can be attributed to subjective responses in part. However, some of these explanations can be eliminated to a large extent due to the evidence available. Poor concentration of subjects can be caused by lack of interest in the experiment, or by tiredness due to the duration of the experiment. Average levels of inconsistency were similar for the technical subjects as for the naïve subjects, and so it seems unlikely, in general, that the subjects were disinterested. It is possible that subjects do become tired, though experiments were limited to 15 minute sessions. Evidence suggests that explanations b) and d) would be the main causes of inconsistencies. It is true that as the variance in dBA between stimuli decreases then the likelihood of having a clear preference between stimuli is reduced. However in this case the stimuli were specifically chosen for their distinct features other than 'level'. The comments of subjects also supports this view, that there were sufficient differences in the noise quality between stimuli for the subjects to make definite judgements in regard to their preference. Working on the theory that to a large extent the subjects are using different criteria for their preferences between stimuli in the same group, then clearly an inconsistent response is perfectly conceivable and does not indicate an invalid answer, but rather supports the idea that different components in the noise do influence a subject's judgement. However, the widespread nature of inconsistencies makes for difficulties in modelling of the objective measures with the subjective responses, since it is not immediately obvious which components in the noise the subjects are basing their preferences upon.

The notion of inconsistencies also causes limitations upon linear regression analysis based upon the total subjective rating of each stimulus. This limitation is not only due to disagreements between subjects. Where inconsistencies exist (for whatever reason), the stated preference between individual stimuli may well contradict the overall subjective rating. Such a contradictions mean that even a perfect correlation of overall subjective ratings with objective measurements could not highlight the feature. This is why Multi-Dimensional Scaling analysis is required, to expose such inter-stimuli preferences.

3.3 Subject disagreement (coefficient of concordance)

The measure of agreement between subjects is known as the Coefficient of Concordance. This measure is not related to the Coefficient of Consistency in it's statistical origins, and concerns purely the overall ranking of stimuli. It is, of course, desirable to have good agreement between subjects so that correlation with the objective model will apply to a large percentage of the population. Where significant disagreement between subjects occurs, this would suggest that no single model (algorithm) could account for the majority of subjective responses. Despite the fact that more consistent subjects are, generally, in greater agreement, (although this is not always the case), there is no evidence of a core of subjects with significantly similar responses. Disagreement between subjects could have similar causes as with subject inconsistencies, and could be seen as a sort of group inconsistency. In this case either the subjects genuinely do disagree, or their disagreement is caused by preferences based upon different criteria. For the case in point the group response matrix and the coefficients of consistency and concordance are shown below in table 1. The power-steering noise a pair comparison was made by 17 subjects on 11 noise stimuli; each stimuli lasting approximately 5 seconds. The group response matrix below was then calculated, denoting a score of 1 for each subject's preference.

Table 1 Group response Matrix

	A	B	C	D	E	F	G	H	I	J	K
A	-	1	0	0	1	2	0	6	0	2	3
B	16	-	13	17	17	16	14	17	15	17	17
C	17	4	-	16	17	16	9	17	16	17	17
D	17	0	1	-	5	8	2	16	9	11	15
E	16	0	0	12	-	10	2	16	9	17	15
F	15	1	1	9	7	-	5	16	1	15	17
G	17	3	8	15	15	12	-	17	17	17	17
H	11	0	0	1	1	1	0	-	0	5	5
I	17	2	1	8	8	16	0	17	-	16	17
J	15	0	0	6	0	2	0	12	1	-	8
K	14	0	0	2	2	0	0	12	0	9	-

Mean coefficient of consistency = 0.96
Coefficient of Concordance = 0.64

3.4 Multi-dimensional scaling (mds)

MDS analysis of subjective response data enables detailed breakdown of the group response matrices such as the case for the power-steering noise (table 1). Individual inter-stimuli preferences are examined as opposed to the group subject preference rating scores. In the ideal case such analysis would expose dimensions in the responses which can be equated to the identified components of noise. Inter-stimuli distances, based upon the normalised scale of preference between stimuli, were calculated and submitted for analysis. Estimates of the individual stimuli co-ordinates were produced based upon the MDS dimensions. The stress levels are a measure of the goodness of fit of the computer MDS model to the original inter-stimuli distances according to the following scale.

Stress value	Quality of solution
0.4	Poor
0.2	Fair
0.1	Good
0.05	Excellent
0.0	Perfect

In this case a solution for two dimensions was found providing a good fit to the real data, with the solution to three dimensions giving only marginal improvements. Multi- dimensional scaling of these results was carried out by considering the distance between the stimuli as a result of the pair comparison scores. It was found that the subject responses would 'fit' comfortably within two dimensions, with little stress in the result. If the result for this is plotted in the two dimensions a natural grouping was discovered amongst the stimuli (figure 3).

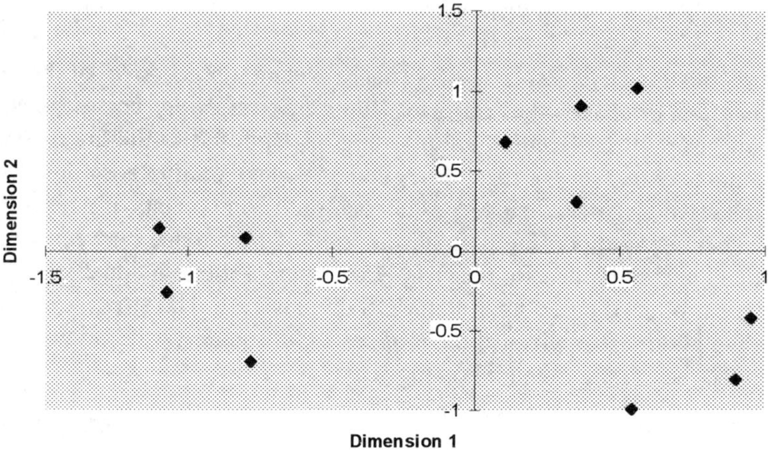

Figure 3. Dimensional Analysis of the Group Response

As a result of MDS analysis, it should be possible to identify the individual components in the noise that pertain to the criteria used by subjects in their evaluation. This is suggested in the in the diagram below.

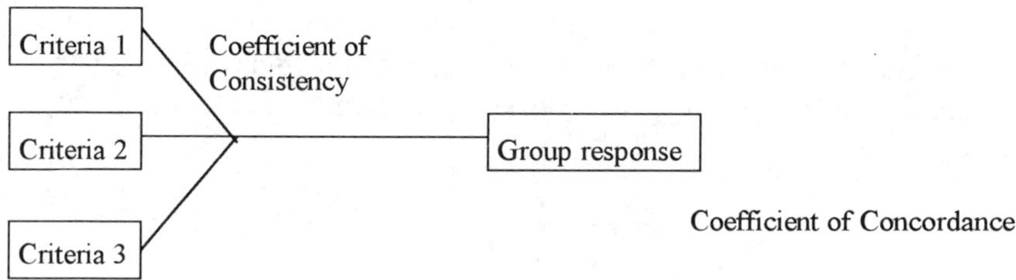

Orthogonal (independent) Components

4. OBJECTIVE ANALYSIS

A number of objective parameter were identified as being key to the subjective issues, though their relative importance and combination were unknown at this stage. Six parameters were found to be important:

- 10th order levels of pump rotation
- 20th order levels of pump rotation
- 30th order levels of pump rotation
- octave band background levels for 10th order of pump rotation
- octave band background levels for 20th order of pump rotation
- octave band background levels for 30th order of pump rotation

Note: all levels A-weighted

The latter 3 parameters provide a measure of the masking effects upon the harmonic components. It is important to note here that not all these 6 parameters are independent of one another; an important consideration in correlation with subject responses. However, the pump speed of rotation used in these experiments was such that the octave bands associated with each order were different.

5. CORRELATION OF OBJECTIVE PARAMETERS WITH SUBJECT RESPONSE

Correlation of these parameters was carried out against the dimensional analysis of the subject response. It quickly showed that all 6 parameters were significant. It also showed that the first dimension in figure 3 correlated well with a combination of 10th and 30th order, whilst the second dimension correlated reasonably well with 20th order. This is consistent with our understanding of the mechanisms of the pump in question, in that the 10th and 30th order sources are generated by the same mechanism and different from that which generates the 20th order. This now proves to be invaluable, since it is potentially possible to change the pump design to improve aspects associated with just one of the dimension. The correlation of these parameters with subject response was further improved by accounting for the background noise of each pump harmonic. This is summarised in figure 4 below.

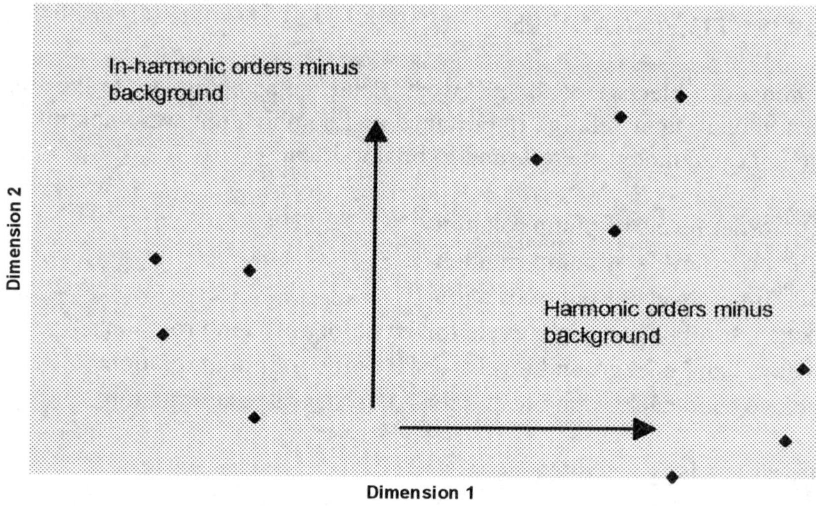

Figure 4. Correlation of objective parameters with subject responses

The correlation coefficients for dimension1 and dimension 2 with the objective parameters above were 0.82, and 0.57 respectively. It now remains to develop an algorithm based upon these objective components that will support the subjective ratings, whilst highlighting the key components (criteria) influencing the subjective assessments.

6. SUMMARY

The issues surrounding subjective appraisal of vehicle interior noise are primarily concerned with subject inconsistencies in response and disagreements between subjects. In many cases the primary explanation for these inconsistencies is a change in the choice of criteria for subjective judgements. It is the case that these phenomena need to be considered as part of any analysis of subject response. Where inconsistencies and disagreements are prevalent the traditional rating schemes are limited in nature, and cannot interpret the results accurately. The discussion above has to some extent shown a methodology by which these inconsistencies can not only be accounted for, but can also be used to identify the key objective parameters influencing the subject responses. It now remains to implement the identified components in a single algorithm that will yield a single value, whilst highlighting the individual component (criteria) that lead to the rating judgement.

REFERENCE

1.   Guilford JP, "Psychometric Methods" McGraw-Hill Series 1954.

Authors addresses

D. Fish
MIRA
Watlingstreet
Nuneaton
Warwichshire CV 10 0TU
United Kingdom

J. Godthelp
TNO Human Factors Institute
Postbus 23
3769 ZG Soesterberg
The Netherlands

H. Happel
Zaïrestraat 53
2622 ES Delft

A.C. Hekstra
TNO Road-Vehicles Research Institute
P.O. Box 6033
2600 JA Delft
The Netherlands

W. Hirschberg
Steyer-Daimler Puch Fahrzeugtechnik
P.O. Box 824
A-8011 Graz
Austria

F. Horkay
Renault S.A.
CTR A2/Service 60502
67 Rue des Bous-Raisins
92508 Rueil-Malmaison
France

Ch. Jung
MAN Nutzfahrzeuge AG
Postfach 500620
D-80976 München
Germany

W. Käppler
X-perience Multimedia Training & System Design GmbH
Wilhelm Levisonstrasse 12
D-53115 Bonn
Germany

R. Kempeneers
Dutch Driver's Licence Authority
P.O. Box 5301
2280 HH Rijswijk
The Netherlands

W. Kiesewetter
Kantweg 3
D-71336 Waiblingen
Germany

W. Klinkner
Mercedes Benz
Abt. EP/KBR
D-70322 Stuttgart
Germany

J. Kohn
Dunlop Tyres SP
Tyres UK Ltd.
Fort Dunlop
Irdington, Birmingham B24 9QT
United Kingdom

D. Kudritzki
Audi AG
Abt. I/EF - 5/drku
D-85045 Ingolstadt
Germany

J.P. Pauwelussen
TNO Road-Vehicles Research Institute
P.O. Box 6033
2600 JA Delft
The Netherlands

B. Peters
VTI- Swedisch Road and Transport Research Institute
S-581 95 Linköping
Sweden

W. Reichelt
Daimler Benz AG
Abt. F1M/FA
D-70546 Stuttgart
Germany

A. Savkoor
Delft University of Technology
Mekelweg 2
OCP-tt
2628 CD Delft
The Netherlands

R. Sharp
School of Mechanical Engineering
Cranfield University
Bedford MK43 0AL
United Kingdom

M. Steiner
Hanflandstrasse 11
D-71364 Winnenden
Germany

P. Stephens
Dunlop Tyres SP
Tyres UK Ltd.
Fort Dunlop
Irdington, Birmingham B24 9QT
United Kingdom

A. de Vos
TNO Human Factors Institute
Postbus 23
3769 ZG Soesterberg
The Netherlands

Index